Go to www.brandysevans.com/free-download to receive
your free guide to LISTEN! Helping Your Child Manage
Their Emotions.

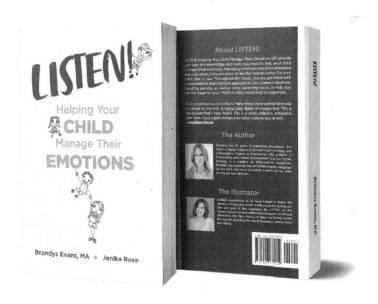

LISTEN!

Helping your

CHILD

manage their

EMOTIONS

BRANDYS EVANS

Illustrated by Jenika Rose

Dedication

This book is dedicated to Tate and Jenika,
my greatest achievements.

Acknowledgements

Thank you to Jenika Rose and Tate Evans for growing with me.

Thank you to my parents, Brent and Barbara, for always believing in me.

Thank you to Dalias Blake for being my personal Neutral.

Thank you to Marianne Stewart for being a strong woman in my life.

Thank you to Amanda Rogers, my exceptional and amazing editor for her insight and support. And thanks to my formatter, Lebanon Raingam for his fantastic work to make this book an enjoyable read.

Thank you to Gary Williams for guiding me through the process and his enthusiastic support.

Thank you to Phi Do for his ability to understand human thought patterns and his willingness to satiate my curious mind.

Thank you to Roxanne Gresham, a great listener!

Thank you Kathleen Cobon and everyone who supported me through the publishing process.

Contents

FOREWORD

This book is about emotions. I provide guidance on how to help your child to manage their emotions. It is my belief that the ability to manage emotions cannot be taught. The management of one's emotions requires nurturance and cultivation in the presence of another human being. In the case of your child and their emotions, that person is you.

Feeling emotions is like stretching. At first, it feels painful. You are tempted to not push into the pain. The brain says, "Stop! I don't like pain." But, you know that a good stretch feels good once you're done. You find that as you breathe and push into the stretch, that the pain starts to fade, and you feel a loosening. The best part is when you have moved into the stretch long enough and you feel a release. Then the stretch is over, and you feel relaxed and at ease.

The same is true for our emotions. When you first meet with emotion, there is a temptation to make it stop or go away (think any childhood tantrums). The brain says, "This is *really* uncomfortable!" However, the more you lean into the emotion, the more the mind starts to settle. You feel an emotional release. The emotion has passed, and you feel more at ease.

This book combines personal and professional experience that makes sense to me and several others I have worked with. Teaching emotion regulation does not make sense to me because the teaching brain is not readily available when a child is emotional. Teaching most often happens before and after the child's emotional experience. It is my belief that this is a source of instilling in children a sense of helplessness and disconnection from themselves. If you want a child to regulate their emotions, then you have to work with the part of the brain that generates emotion. This is what this book is about.

To help you better understand your child's emotional experience, I break it down for you. In the first section, I will talk about the parts of the brain that are players in the game of emotion regulation. In the second section, I break down the experience of emotion with insight that makes sense.

In the third section, I share how to nurture and cultivate emotion regulation in your child. In the fourth section, I offer practical applications in point form for a brief overview regarding common situations faced by parents. As a bonus, I added some parenting hacks, or tools that help you set the stage for your child's healthy emotional growth.

This book is the culmination of the two greatest nurturers and cultivators in my world, Jenika Rose and Tate Evans. Enjoy!!

"The most important childhood predictor of adult satisfaction is the child's emotional health, followed by the child's conduct. The least powerful predictor is the child's intellectual development."

Layard, R., Clark, A. E., Cornaglia, F., Powdthavee, N., & Vernoit, J. (2014). What predicts a successful life? A life-course model of well-being. *Economic journal (London, England)*, *124(580)*, F720–F738. doi:10.1111/ecoj.12170

PART A:
THE BRAIN

The brain can be your greatest ally when raising your child. It can also be your greatest enemy. Either way, the brain provides many of the answers that you've been searching for. Understanding the way that the brain works will help you to understand your child, as well as help you to understand why he behaves the way that he does.

Your child's brain is like his own personal sports team. The game he is playing is the game of life (no, not the boardgame). The trophy, the banner, and the celebration cup are what he achieves when he feels good about himself.

Your child's team needs a coach. That coach is you. The team cannot succeed without you. The players need training. They need to build strength and stamina and they need direction on how to perform their role on the team.

Your child's team has to work together to experience success. When the team does not play well together, your child will experience a setback. The result is a child that does not feel good about himself. So, you want the team to play well together. You want your child to feel good about himself. You want him to feel strong, resilient and capable.

Have you ever coached your child's sports team? Being your child's coach may be one of the most important investments that you ever make. By this, I do not mean their soccer, basketball, or baseball team. I mean the coach for your child's brain, for Team Brain.

Understanding Team Brain, the team members, their positions, and having access to the playbook will provide you with the information you need to effectively coach. You can lead this team to win the championship. The championship is your child feeling good about himself.

So, let's get going. Introducing, Team Brain.

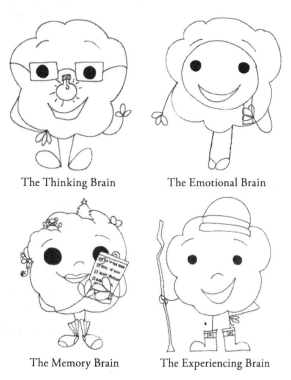

The Thinking Brain   The Emotional Brain

The Memory Brain   The Experiencing Brain

CHAPTER 1:
The Thinking Brain

"When you are a bear of very little brain, and you think things, you sometimes find that a thing which seemed very thingish inside you is quite different when it gets out into the open and has other people looking at it."
- WINNIE-THE-POOH

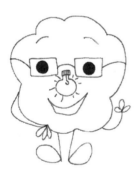

Title: The Thinking Brain
- Rational
- Logical
- Analytical
- Makes good decisions

W e are intelligent beings, for the most part. We are creative. We come up with new ideas, make plans, and work towards our goals. Much of the work involved in this task-oriented process comes from our Thinking Brain.

The Thinking Brain is just beginning the process of growth when a child is born. The Thinking Brain will undergo 24 years of construction and reconstruction until it has reached full maturity.

The Thinking Brain is like the Captain of the team. Not necessarily because it is the best, but because it is a leader. The Thinking Brain likes to put goals into action. It likes to make things happen. It uses its intelligence to think, to be rational, and to make well thought out decisions to move the team in a positive direction.

Disney's on-screen rendition of *The Jungle Book (2016)* depicts an example of the Thinking Brain in action. Abandoned in the jungle and raised by wolves, Mowgli journeys to a man village. Mowgli requires protection from a Tiger that hunts man out of revenge for a man inflicted wound.

Mowgli disregards the warning of his wise animal escorts. The warning is to refrain from human-like behaviour for his protection. Acting human would draw attention to the man-cub and alert the tiger of his whereabouts.

Mowgli resisted and instead followed his instinct to set goals, to be creative, and to problem solve. His goals were to meet his need for food, shelter, and protection. His behaviour supported his needs, disregarding what others thought was best for him.

We move forward towards attainable goals for our growth and expansion. We meet our goals when our Thinking Brain is well functioning.

In contrast, the Thinking Brain stops working when the Emotional Brain turns on. It's like in football where you have an offensive team and a defensive team. These two teams do not play on the field at the same time, (well, not if they are on the same team).

When the offense is playing, the defense is on the sidelines waiting for the chance to do what they are trained to do. And, vice versa. When the defense is on the field, the offense is taking a rest.

Emotions are our defense and the Emotional Brain is the defensive team. Strong emotional experiences shut off the Thinking Brain, sending the Thinking Brain to the sidelines. The Emotional Brain steps in to do its job.

In other words, when we feel emotion, our Thinking Brain shuts off and stops working. When this happens, your child can't think clearly. She can't problem solve, she can't verbalize, and she can't make sense of the situation. She feels out of control.

So, teaching your child how to respond when they are emotional is ineffective. The Thinking Brain loves to learn and to hold new and helpful information. But, this part of the brain is not accessible when your child is emotional. The Thinking Brain is on the sidelines. Your child needs help tending to her emotions before she can apply the calming tools that have been taught to her.

A father said it best when he shared his experience with anger management classes. He acknowledged his appreciation for the tools and techniques presented to help manage his anger. "It would be nice if they actually worked when you're angry!" was his honest evaluation of the process.

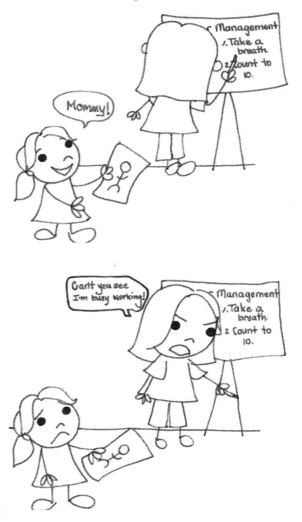

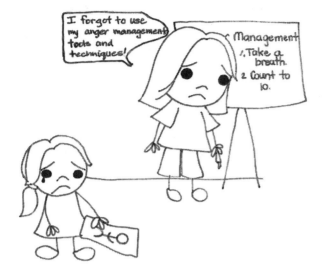

The Thinking Brain is available for learning. It is more than happy to generate learned tools for the sake of problem solving. But this is successful if there is no interference from the Emotional Brain.

You can teach your child skills to regulate emotion. But, your child's ability to control herself will not come from what you teach her. Her ability to manage her behaviour and her emotions will come from the way you interact with her emotions.

Tools and techniques do not work if the Thinking Brain is shut off. So why train a team in a position that they won't ever play? It can help with managing emotion, but not until your child is much older. Your team will not be successful. Your child will not be able to control her emotions if you ask the thinking brain to do the Emotional Brain's job.

The Thinking Brain is there to help your child problem solve and to meet goals. Once the Emotional Brain's job is done (and you are there to help), the Emotional Brain will leave the playing field and the Thinking Brain can come back on the field and get to work.

If you want to win the game, you must place the most effective players on your team in their proper position. You need to play the defensive team when the team is under threat and play the offense team when it's time to advance. You must use the Thinking Brain for growth and your Emotional Brain to manage emotions.

CHAPTER 2:
The Emotional Brain

"How do you spell love Pooh?"
-PIGLET

"You don't spell it, you feel it."
-WINNIE-THE-POOH

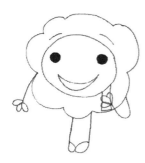 **Title: The Emotional Brain**
- Irrational
- Illogical
- Reactive
- Makes rash decisions

Your child is an emotional being. Emotion is essential for his survival. Emotion communicates what is going on inside of him. For example, joy communicates pleasure, sadness communicates pain.

The Emotional Brain is all ready to go when a child is born. Your child's world will communicate through emotion for many years to come, while the Thinking Brain slowly develops.

The Emotional Brain is the defender. This is the part of the brain that is there to protect the team from danger. The Emotional Brain deals with whatever is coming up in the moment. He does not care whatever else may be going on. His primary purpose is to ensure the safety and survival of the team by putting forth a strong fight. He is incessant and will fight and defend until he knows that everything is going to be okay.

The Emotional Brain also communicates need. Think about a time that your child was emotional. Did you know what your child was communicating? Has your child ever thrown a tantrum because they wanted something, and you said "No"?

I used to think that these extreme expressions came from children of pushover parents. That was, until I had the experience myself.

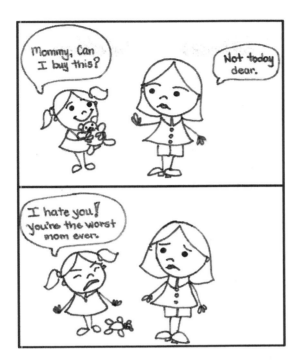

What I learned was that my child was communicating a need. Her young mind fully believed that what she *wanted* was a *need*, i.e. "I *have* to have this." When I did not give in to what she *wanted*, she felt intense discomfort. Her emotional response communicated desperation (not a reflection of her personality). Her Emotional Brain was defending her position.

An emotional child is an activated child. A child will become activated when a *perceived* need is not met. You've experienced this, the screaming, yelling, or demanding that drives you nuts. This means, for the most part, that your child's Thinking Brain has turned off. Unbridled emotion becomes the communicator of the moment, which is often shown through undesirable behaviour.

As parents, we often look at behaviour as the problem. It's our child's emotionally driven behaviour that affects us. It makes us feel emotional and it affects our own behaviour.

Have you ever noticed how often you use emotion when dealing with your child (i.e. raise your voice, get defensive, argue, demand)? We get caught up in the rush of the moment, overcome by discomfort, fear of judgement, or our own limitations. Our Emotional Brain is on the defense as well. We want that uncomfortable feeling inside of us to go away. We want the behaviour to stop.

But wait!

Your child's behaviour is not the source of the problem. The root of the problem is the intense discomfort felt in the moment.

An activated emotional brain means that your child is not rational or logical. Your child cannot make a clear decision or solve a problem. Your child struggles to find the words to describe what he is experiencing.

The Emotional Brain, also known as the amygdala, is the part of the brain that drives your child's intense behaviour. His behaviour is communicating a need. Your job is to assess the difference between need and want and to set boundaries for your child.

Healthy boundary setting helps your child to develop the ability to tolerate uncomfortable emotions. Eventually, he will manage his own emotional state and his behaviour.

Your job is to also identify other messages from the Emotional Brain. When you acknowledge the message, the Emotional Brain's job is done. Your child no longer needs their defensive team. When the Emotional Brain has settled, your child will return to clarity of thought. The Thinking Brain can come back on the field and start to work towards success.

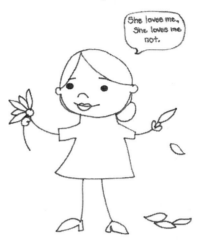

Remember this when you hear your child say that they hate you and that you're an awful parent.

This is a reflection of how your child is feeling about *himself*. This translates to,

"Help me! I am out of control and I can't do this alone."

Your child is not born with the ability to regulate his emo-

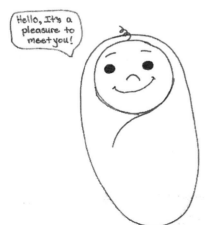

tions. If this were the case, your child would have had a different entrance into the world.

When your child is emotional, their body is in a state of survival. Your child needs you to hear him in this moment, to hear what his body is communicating. How you respond to his emotions will impact his ability to manage them.

Listening is crucial, as an emotional reaction is more than what you see. Listening is more about what you feel. When you feel the impact of your child's emotions, your own system will want to make this stop. You must *listen* to both yourself *and* to your child to manage the emotions from both of you.

Listening means attuning to the physiological changes that occur when your child is activated. Managing these activated moments is how you cultivate emotional regulation in your child. This starts with you not engaging with your child's emotional response.

To help your child manage his emotions, you have to work with the Emotional Brain. You must train the defensive team and let the team do its job. Its job is to respond, not react. To not flinch and be with the emotion until it passes.

This is where a child learns to manage his emotions. When he experiences tolerance for the emotion. When he can be with the activated experience until it passes. This is how he manages his emotions, and improves every single time he gets a chance to play on the field.

Success is a child that can manage his emotions and his behaviour. The result is a child that feels incredible about himself.

CHAPTER 3:
The Memory Brain

"I was so busy being upset that I forgot to be happy."
-EEYORE

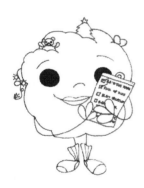

Title: The Memory Brain
- Storage
- Emotional Remembering

We are intelligent. The Thinking Brain is our captain.

Memory plays an essential role in your child's development. Growth and development is her destiny. Memory allows the storage of information from your child's past to influence what she does in the present and to drive her towards her future. Without memory, she would not be able to set goals, to make plans, or to problem solve.

The Memory Brain is like an assistant coach. It keeps all the data and helps assist in decision making for the success of the team. The Memory Brain provides reminders of past experiences, especially uncomfortable or threatening ones.

Intense emotional experiences create strong memories. Whether positive or negative, these memories become seared in our heart and mind.

For example, I will never forget that day in grade eight when I was late for school. I was trying to shed off my good girl image with the help of a nonchalant attitude towards school tardiness.

While using my locker as a fast food window for an English binder and writing utensils, I heard it! The enticing sound of John Braithwaite's Mod style footwear echoed "clunk...ching... clunk...ching!" as he walked down the hallway. I felt my heart beat faster and faster, like a military grade machine gun as the sound grew louder and louder.

He was getting closer. "I've got to play this cool!" were the only words I could make sense of in my flustered mind.

Sensing his tall, masculine body behind me, I slowly closed my locker door and carefully turned around. Time stopped. He placed his hands on either side of my face, leaned in and gave me my first kiss ever. He then walked away without saying a word.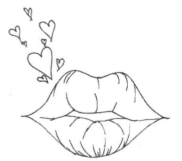

OH! MY! GOODNESS!

My legs went weak and my insides turned to mush as my lips experienced that exhilarating moment.

My children have heard this story at nauseam. Why? Because it had such a significant impact on me. The memory is forever in my brain because *it was emotional.* It was more than a first kiss. That moment followed months of anticipation, flirtation, and youthful feminine emotions.

Anytime I hear the words *first kiss*, the above memory pops into my brain. This memory is not an account of the story that unfolded, but a deep and lasting emotional *experience* that is seared into my mind. The emotion that I felt in that moment of time became the source of the memory.

The Memory Brain, or the hippocampus, is a filing system. It is the storage centre for emotional memories. Your child's Emotional Brain and Memory Brain work together to process all the information that comes into your child's world.

The Memory Brain provides reminders of times when your child felt uncomfortable. Much like having a performance analysis constantly available. This results in a fast and efficient response time for the safety of your child.

When the Emotional Brain is on the playing field, the Memory Brain sets the play in motion. It reminds the Emotional Brain of past encounters so the Emotional Brain can do its job. Its job is to protect and preserve the team. And when that job is done, the Thinking Brain takes over and can move the team towards success.

Your child's mind pays particular attention to moments when she needs to react. A reaction occurs in a split second for the sake of her preservation. This happens long before she has the capacity to think.

Have you ever seen your child reactive, or what you may call over-reactive? Have you told your child to calm down, to relax, or to "stop it"? Does your child struggle to let go or move on?

If your experience is much like my own, it doesn't work very well, does it?

Have *you* ever tried that yourself? *Letting go* is not that easy. It rarely works because there is emotional content stuck to the memory like a super-bonded crazy glue. The memory probably got there in the first place during a time you felt discomfort.

The brain does not like uncomfortable feelings. So, your child's Memory Brain vividly stores any moment of discomfort. All her efforts become focused on avoiding that feeling. The Emotional Brain goes on the defensive to solve uncomfortable situations, i.e. the tantrum. Memory acts as a protector. But, it can also get in the way.

Stored emotional memories from the past can get in the way of living today. Attending to emotion, such as saying, "Looks like you are really scared today!" can help The Memory Brain work through and release stored emotional responses. Setting healthy boundaries helps the assistant coach to learn new skills that are less reactive and more productive. And move the team towards success.

And before we end this chapter, are you wondering how the memory of an amazing first kiss is needed for survival? Well, an amazing kiss can contribute to the preservation of our species... just saying ;)!

CHAPTER 4:
The Experiencing Brain

"Sometimes the smallest things can take up the biggest room in your heart."
- WINNIE-THE-POOH

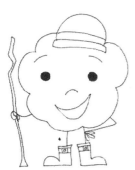

Title: The Experiencing Brain
- Ties it all together
- Knows the moment well

Experience can be a master teacher. We learn from our experiences or we learn from the experiences of others. The more we experience the more we learn. The more we learn, the more we know, and the more we know the more resources we have to achieve our goals.

The Experiencing Brain is the Captain of the team. It can see the big picture and brings it all together.

Experience is not only an external occurrence. Underneath our skin is an array of experiences taking place every second of the day. This includes the experience of your body's complex system of protection.

For example, you know that moment when your child seems off? You can sense that something is not right. You have so much to get done and your child seems intent on distracting you.

This powerful force draws you in. Your attempts to redirect your child's energy away from you proves futile. In that moment you think, "If I ignore this, it will pass." But this does not work. The more you try to redirect your child, the more energy he puts into garnering your attention.

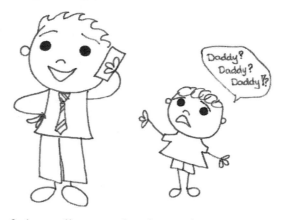

You can feel it well up inside of you, that mounting pressure that is ready to burst at any moment. This is what you are *experiencing*.

Your child can feel this. He can *sense* this. And, it creates a feeling of discomfort. He wants this feeling to go away. He continues to persist at getting your undivided attention to make him feel better. He needs your attention for the discomfort to go away. This is what your child is *experiencing*.

Your response to your child influences his ability to manage this discomfort. You feel the energy created by your body's activated state. Your child experiences the energy of their own activated state. And then, this experience is felt between the two of you.

In every moment, your child lives an experience deep within himself. The Experiencing Brain, or the insular cortex, combines everything that is going on outside and inside your child and generates the *experience*.

When your child's body needs to do something, there is a hormonal surge. A sensation results in the body that communicates what is happening. In this moment, your child experiences a physiological change. This may include sensations such as a pounding heart, nausea, shaking, or tightness in the chest or head.

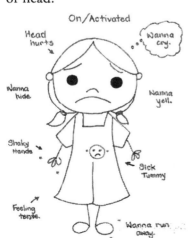

This sensory experience happens on many different levels. Your child may or may not be aware that this is happening. Regardless, his *behaviour* will communicate to you what is going on. A quiet and withdrawn child is internalizing the experience. And, children that externalize are hard to miss!

Your child's behaviour is a symptom of what is happening in the moment. His behaviour is not the entire story of what your child is *experiencing*. We often see behaviour as the issue, when it is only a part of the story.

Take, for example, a meltdown in the car. Your child may freak out because they did not get a snack or screen time that they were hoping for. You're bothered by the behaviour. Exhausted, you act on their behaviour and lecture or reprimand his actions. What you did not do was consider the stress that your child was under after the affairs of his day.

Instead of reacting, you say, "Sounds like you have had a rough day", "I can see how angry/sad/nervous you are" and wait. Just listen. Listen to the space. Suspend the part where you need to make you feel better. Notice how tending to your child's emotional needs actually results in a calmer space. See how everyone starts to feel more grounded and how problem solving happens naturally.

Keep in mind that this does not mean that you condone the behaviour. It's just that reprimands or lectures don't help the situation. They actually make matters worse. When you do this, your behaviour communicates that your child needs to take care of you. You communicate that taking care of your own discomfort was more important than being there to help her take care of her own.

Challenging behaviour directly affects you. Yet, it is more to do with the raw *experience* of a child. A child does not know how to communicate this with their words.

You expect your child to explain himself and correct his behaviour even though adults have a hard enough time doing either of these things. Unfortunately, your child's Thinking Brain is not yet developed enough to do the job. Plus, his Thinking Brain is most likely not working at all if your child is already quite emotional.

Your child's behaviour is less likely to have anything to do with the snack or the screen time. The behaviour is more likely to do with something that happened earlier in the day, the week, or the year. Difficulties can stem from anything such as peers, schoolwork, or family conflict - or all the above combined! And, your child wants you there to help him through the process.

Your child cannot handle his emotions on his own. He needs you to identify them, be with them, and allow them to move through him. This is how you help his emotional energy to release and have less of a negative effect on anyone involved. He needs you.

Have you ever asked yourself, "Why does my child behave so 'poorly' with me and not others?" For the most part, you will be an innocent bystander in your child's world of dysregulation. You will be the dumping ground for what your child is *experiencing*.

You cannot take this as a personal attack. Instead, use this as a sign of how much your child needs you. When your child is not with you, they have to be on good behaviour for the sake of fitting in. When your child is with you, he will work through a spectrum of emotional experiences. He needs to do this to grow. He needs *you* to grow.

A child often acts out more so with the person that they feel most connected to. It's within this connection that your child develops his ability to manage his emotions.

Children need an adult to nurture and cultivate this life skill. It is in the presence of your caring and attention that your child will cultivate the ability to manage their emotions. You must be able to manage the energy that arises from your child. In this space, your child will develop the ability to manage himself.

When you view your child's reactions as their *experience*, you have compassion and understand the need for your child to grow. You have patience with the experience, especially when it is difficult. When you can hear your child, you can help your child to hear himself. This is the foundation of your child managing their emotions.

PART B: EMOTION

We live in a world that values thought. *Think before you speak. Your thoughts control your actions.* Think positively to rid yourself of negativity.

Sounds like a good plan, right?

So then, why is it so hard to keep positive? Because! Thought is designed to problem solve, not to make us *feel* better.

Thoughts are like paving a road. The more you think about a thought, the more road you pave. Sometimes we clear land to pave new roads. And other times, we pave over old roads, such as the cobblestone roads in older cities.

Cobblestone roads are like our emotions. You either excavate the stones and prepare the road for new pavement, or you pave over the cobblestones. As the new road wears and tears, you are exposed to earth or cobblestone underneath.

When exposed to earth, a pothole forms. Road maintenance comes to repair the road for your safe driving. When exposed to cobblestone, the road is often left unattended. History shows its face and you are left driving over a combination of paved road and cobblestone road, bumpy and uncomfortable.

When you do not remove your cobblestones, or your past emotions, they lie in wait. They wait until enough wear and tear occurs on your life, and then they show through.

Why?

Because emotions are more powerful than thoughts. This is why it is hard to simply *let go* or *just move on*. Because there is cobblestone underneath the pavement. There are emotions stored within that are keeping you safe, keeping your child safe.

In order to allow thought to do its job, you first must attend to the emotion. To attend to the emotion, it would help if you understood what exactly emotion is. In this section, I break it down to answer the question, "What is emotion?" in the way the answer makes sense to me.

CHAPTER 5:

What is an Emotion?

I'm so happy, I could bounce"
- TIGGER

It's finally here. That time of day that you have been long-ing for. The nighttime routine is complete, your child is in bed, and you finally sit down for a moment of peace. "Daddy, I need you!" rings through your ears and startles your body. Your child wants you, again!

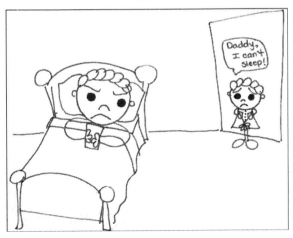

"Go away. I need a moment to be alone!" is what you would like to say. You refrain (or not) and go about the never-ending exhausting battle of getting your child off to bed. If this is not you, please don't rub it in! For those that can relate, it's frustrating. It's *emotional*.

Here is a formula for emotion:

Stimulus/Thought + Physiological Response + Assessment of the Situation = Emotion

For example:

Hearing Your Child's Voice + Internal Jolt + Child Not in Bed Standing at Your Door = Anger/Frustration

Stimulus

Your child's mind is like the best security system ever used in a Mission Impossible movie. Every facet of your child is alert and aware of their surroundings at all times. Her brain is registering everything that goes on around her. This provides the information necessary for growth, development, and safety.

It also provides the information that will keep her safe.

We learn about our surroundings through stimuli, or messages from the environment, that comes in through our senses. The following are eight senses that provide information to your child's mind on a daily basis.

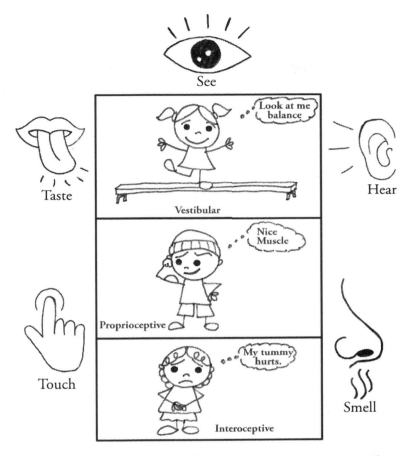

Your child has all these different messages coming into her mind that help her determine what she will do in any given moment.

Thought

What do you think comes first, thought or emotion?

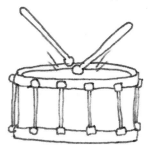

The answer is...both.

Thought can be generated at any given moment. Close your eyes and block out the world, and you will start thinking about all kinds of things. Your child can generate thoughts from information that is already stored within the mind, especially since your child's mind is extremely creative.

Emotion precedes thought after alarming messages come into the brain. Your child may feel discomfort from having to speak in front of the class. The information coming from the senses filters through the Emotional Brain before reaching the Thinking Brain. When the message is activating, the Emotional Brain generates energy because the body needs to do something.

First, her body becomes activated. Then her stomach feels queasy, her body shakes, and her head feels tight. She may or may not be aware of what is happening. Then thoughts begin, "I hate school!"

Physiological Response

Stress! Your child knows it well. Stress is when your child's mind receives a message that needs a reaction. Peers, family dynamics, school, extracurricular activities, and academics are potential stressors.

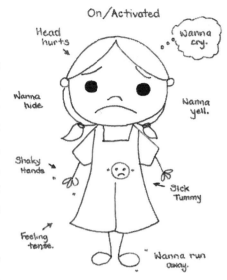

Stress produces energy in your child's body. This instantaneous surge of energy occurs before your child can even begin to think or reflect on the situation. There are changes happening inside your child.

For example, this is how my daughter ended up in a time out on her first day of kindergarten. During afternoon circle time, a boy repeatedly was falling asleep and landing in her lap. After multiple attempts to re-position her classmate, she hit him.

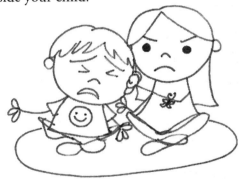

Yes, my daughter got in trouble on her first day of kindergarten for trying to keep a boy's head out of her lap!

My daughter has always been a protector of her space and the imposition of a stranger was activating a defense within her. She reacted out of frustration and a need to protect herself. She did not reflect and consider the consequences. She reacted based on the energy that was created within her and what her 5-year-old brain believed needed to happen in the moment.

This happens all the time for your child. Your child's responses will be reactionary until she cultivates the ability to understand these internal messages. Once she can tolerate this sensation, she will increase her ability to manage her emotions.

Assessment of the situation

Your child's mind is constantly taking inventory of her surroundings. What is happening in your child's surroundings influences what she is feeling.

Let's use Sam as an example. Sam is an energetic and determined 6-year-old. Sam loves to play soccer during recess. And, he prefers to do this with the older boys.

One day, one of the older boys stopped Sam from playing with the group. This did not go over well with the tenacious first grader. He believed that he was good enough to join the older crew. So, Sam kicked the fifth grader while offering an evaluation of the student's character.

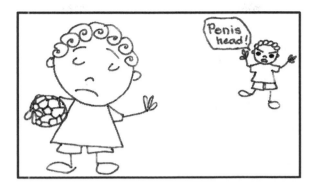

Who got in trouble? Sam, of course. Was Sam confused? Yes!

Sam did not see a problem with his behaviour because according to his six-year-old mind, the fifth grader was in the wrong. The older boy was not being fair, and fairness is the law when you're six.

Was Sam able to control his anger? No. Was the behaviour acceptable? Of course not. Sam got in trouble and had to stay in the classroom for two days during his lunch hour.

Was that an appropriate response to the child's behaviour? I would argue that it was not. I believe that the purpose of the consequence was to *teach* Sam that his behaviour was not acceptable. The desired result was that Sam would make different choices in future situations.

Is this what Sam *learned*? Maybe. Integrated? No! Sam *experienced* that he will lose out if he kicks and calls names. Sam *learned* that he will be punished for speaking up. And, Sam will have *integrated* that he is somehow defective. Though, this will not sit well with Sam, as the tenacious part of him believes that he is of great value.

You see, at the time of the incident, Sam used his best six-year-old resources to handle the situation. He was told that he could not join the game. This upset him. His assessment of the situation was that this was wrong. He believed in his ability. He believed he deserved a chance. So, the surge of energy from his unbridled six-year-old brain was put to good use.

Remember, the Emotional Brain is not verbal and it's there to defend the individual. Sam's fragile and innocent assessment of the situation was that he needed to stand-up for himself. So, kicking the older child would have been the natural solution for this emotionally charged six-year-old.

Standing up to an older boy takes strength, it takes courage. But Sam's consequence communicated that his *strength* was punishable. That *he* is the problem. Generally speaking, children are not born into the world thinking that they are a problem. They learn this through interactions with other individuals.

Sam *experienced* that his ability to advocate and *speak up* for himself was rejected. The result is a child that begins to feel shame, shame about being who he is.

We will talk more about the effect of misreading your child's behaviour. We will also talk more about what to do with the behaviour that is not okay, while helping your child to grow and feel good about himself. For now, we used Sam as an example of how your child's behaviour or emotional response is influenced in the moment.

Did you know that nervousness and excitement are exactly the same emotions going on inside your child? Two children can be *feeling* exactly the same thing on the first day of school, such as a nauseous tummy and low appetite. But, one child is scared because they feel safer when they are close to mom. The other child is feeling excitement because they have been bored all summer and are desperate to get back into the school routine.

Awareness of what is going on around your child will help you understand their emotionally charged behaviour.

Emotional Assignment

Emotion is the summation of thought/stimuli, the changes felt within our body, and how we make sense of that in the moment. Emotion comes from a non-verbal space. Your child *feels* emotion.

But, our Thinking Brain likes to make sense of things. We want to put a word to the *experience*. We want an explanation for *why* our child is *emoting*; we want to know what she is *feeling*.

We use *feeling* words to describe this *experience*.

Fear in a dark bedroom + body freezes + alone and it's dark
= SCARED

Birthday presents + body shakes + it's her birthday
= EXCITED

Helping your child manage their emotions will include knowing what emotions are out there.

The following are considered basic emotions. Your child *experiences* one or more of these emotions on a daily basis.

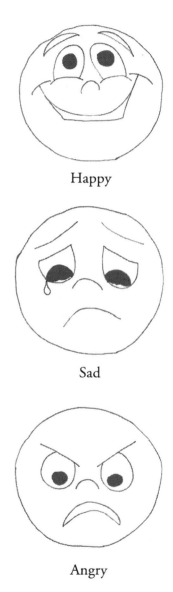

Happy

Sad

Angry

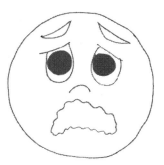

Afraid

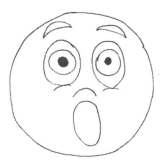

Surprised

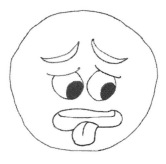

Disgust

These emotions can be felt at varying degrees of intensity.

	Little	**Middle**	**Big**
Joy	Happy	Delighted	Excited
Fear	Nervous	Afraid	Terror
Anger	Bothered	Angry	Furious
Sad	Sad	Low	Miserable
Disgusted	Disgust	Abhorrence	Loathing
Surprised	Surprised	Shocked	Alarmed

And they can also be complex.

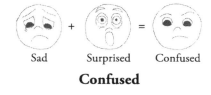

Sad　　　Surprised　　Confused

Confused

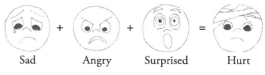

Sad　　　Angry　　Surprised　　Hurt

Hurt

Your child's experience of emotion is subjective. It's like a snowflake. No two snowflakes are alike. No two children respond exactly the same way to a situation.

How your child responds to a situation is neither good nor bad. Emotion does not have morality. It's a part of us, like breathing or sleeping. It just happens.

Take anger, for example. Anger is a pure emotion.

The energy that comes from the emotional *experience* is a motivator to make something happen. It's a good thing. And *you* need to *listen* to what is communicated.

Your child's emotion becomes an issue when it feels bigger than you. Her emotion is communicating, and you feel discomfort. How you manage this discomfort will determine how your child manages her emotions. Identifying the emotion you are feeling will help to stabilize you. Identifying the emotion your child is feeling will help to redirect her raw energy.

Identifying the emotion that your child is feeling is part of the path to success. "You look sad", "You feel embarrassed" are phrases that identify what you sense is happening.

It helps your child to connect to what she is *experiencing* as you put a word to what is happening within her. It helps your child to know that you are trying to understand her. The fact that you are *trying* to understand **powerfully** communicates to your child that she is invaluable. These are all key components of helping your child to manage her emotions.

When your child feels understood, she feels like you care about her success. And successful guidance of emotion results in feeling good about yourself. Even better, successful guidance results in desirable behaviours.

So, successful guidance of your child's emotions will result in a child that feels good about herself and conducts herself respectfully. Isn't that what we want?

When you're there to support your child through their emotional experiences, it brings a feeling of connection. Your child feels more connected to you and your child feels more connected to herself. She feels stronger about herself. She feels motivated to explore and to take on the world.

Emotion is energy. It is the culmination of the body's activated state. It is a motivator and it drives our behaviour.

Hold Slip

Parkgate Branch
31/03/23 11:40AM

Listen! : helping your child manage
their emotions /
33141030896990

ARAYA CERDAS, DIANA

CHAPTER 6:
Behaviour

"Weeds are flowers too, once you get to know them."
- EEYORE

What we don't realize is that *our* emotional state directly impacts our child's behaviour. When our boundaries are not well established, our emotional state affects our children. We tend to blame them for our own emotional moments, especially when everyone is stressed out.

We want challenging moments to dissipate and demand changes in behaviour. This tends to backfire because we use our child's behaviour as the gauge for our own emotional response. We entice the moment and make them take blame.

But, behaviour can be a miscommunication if we don't know how to listen to what our child's body is communicating. When your child is rude and abrupt, your initial reaction may be to challenge the behaviour.

If you take a step back and listen, to hear the activated body, you may hear something more. You may see that the child is tired, or is overwhelmed by the workload at school, or an activity with a peer just fell through.

We don't always know the reason why our child is emotional. What we do know is that an emotional child is trying to meet a need. Not to misbehave or give attitude.

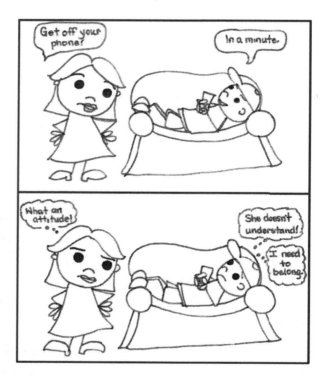

Have you ever wanted to change your child's behaviour? If your answer is yes, you're not alone. Whatever your child is doing in that moment was unnecessary or unwanted.

If the behaviour went away, that would solve your problems, right? Wrong!

Have you considered that your child's behaviour is not the source of the problem? There's always a motivator driving the behaviour. And it may not be as plain as you think.

Behaviour is a symptom.

As parents, we get caught up in our children's behaviours. Behaviours are *in your face*, especially the ones that you don't want to be there. We focus on *changing* these behaviours. Sometimes this is for the good of the child or the good of the situation. Other times, it is for selfish reasons alone.

There are many sources out there that offer how to *fix* your child's behaviour. I've had workbooks in my office to help children *change* unwanted behaviours. After reviewing the contents, this didn't make sense to me.

My argument is that behaviour is not the problem. Behaviour is the symptom. Focusing on changing behaviour misses the point. When you focus on changing behaviour, you tell your child that you are not interested in *him*. You are not interested in understanding him. Nor, do you have the strength to help him in the journey of understanding himself.

This disinterest often stems from your own selfishness. When your child is rude, you want to make that stop. You want an apology, an explanation.

However, what your child needs is for you to listen. To identify the emotion, such as "Sounds like you are feeling upset." If you were to do this, your child would eventually calm and see you as a safe haven.

Unfortunately, what is more common is to continue with punishing the behaviour. After all, you do work your tail off to feed, clothe, shelter and drive your child **everywhere**. Don't you deserve a bit more *respect!*?

See what I mean about selfish? You can get caught up in the behaviour instead of supporting where the behaviour came from.

Trust me, your child does not want to upset you. It may seem that is the intention, but any test of your willpower is a subconscious test to see how **strong** you are. The test is, are you strong enough to withstand being pulled into your child's chaos? Your child needs you to pass that test. Because that is what your child needs to grow their own regulation system.

When your focus is on changing your child's behaviour, you are interested in making him conform to a way of being that *you* think is better. Instead, what helps behaviour is when you first *listen* to what the behaviour is communicating.

When your focus is on the behaviour, your child feels misunderstood. This translates to a sense of shame. Your child begins to feel like something is wrong with him. He feels that he is somehow defective.

But this is confusing for your child, as I believe that we are programmed to think we are pretty awesome! This contradiction creates discomfort. This can manifest as anger, sadness, embarrassment, anxiety, depression, and challenging behaviours. So, he begins to act like he is defective.

This is the last thing you want. But you cannot change the behaviour alone. How comfortable are you with others trying to change you? If your child's behaviour is your focus, your child will feel unaccepted, misunderstood, even frustrated.

Your child does not want to be *changed*. He wants to be understood. To be guided in who he is. To be nurtured. This is how he connects to himself. This is how he becomes his best self.

To feel confident and strong, what your child needs is for you to *listen*. Listening means that you see through the behaviour. Listening says that you can be patient and curious about where the behaviour is coming from.

Listening says that you care enough to not get pulled into the chaos that affects your child. When you do not get pulled into your child's chaos, you communicate that you are strong enough to care for the both of you. You communicate that you are capable to guide your child in developing the ability to manage his emotions.

There is a more effective way to foster healthy behaviour in your child. Healthy behaviour is the result of being able to manage one's own emotions. Your child cannot do this alone. He needs you.

Strength is your ability to manage your own emotions in the presence of your child. When you manage your emotions, your child grows. When his behaviour does not set you off, you help him to develop his own system of emotional management.

Your child needs to feel safe in your presence. This feeling happens when you do *not* become reactive to your child's difficult behaviour. Your job is to remain NEUTRAL.

You actually don't need to work so hard at changing your child's challenging behaviours. When you support your child through the emotional process, the behaviour will correct itself.

The strongest desire of a child before the age of 12 is to please those they are connected to him. The strongest desire for a child after the age of 12 is to gain their approval. So, children do not *want* to behave *badly*. This often is a cry for help, for support as they grow in learning how to manage their emotions.

Working with your child becomes easier when you understand the purpose of behaviour. Behaviour is the communicator.

When the Emotional Brain is active, the Thinking Brain is not working. Children struggle to express what they are experiencing. Adults have a hard-enough time expressing what they are experiencing,

SO WHY DO WE EXPECT CHILDREN TO DO THIS?!

If a child is misbehaving, there is a reason. The reason is generally not a problem *with* the child but *within* the child. Children don't want to misbehave. They want to please you and they want your acceptance.

As parents, we must reprogram *our* mind to see behaviour as a communication tool. We need to stop using behaviour as evidence to label our children.

Behaviours that identify children as difficult can be misunderstood. If you look closer, you can see how the difficulty has arisen.

Take ADHD for example. I have many children that have come into my office with a diagnosis, or pending diagnosis of ADHD. For the majority of these children, when you look at their Psychoeducational Assessment, there is either a learning disability or some area of their learning profile is compromised. The way these children learn is different, and this causes an immense amount of stress deep within the child.

So, guess what happens when you put a child into a classroom that cannot learn like the rest of the students? These children struggle socially. They struggle to focus. They feel stress, or extra energy in their body which needs to be expressed somehow. And a lot of these *behaviours* come from feeling different!

One of our greatest needs is for belonging. So, one of our greatest fears is to be different. Imagine the stress of feeling different every single day! Especially in a world where you are misunderstood. The result is a child that is overreactive or under reactive, attentive, hyperactive, impulsive.

The behaviour then becomes attributed to the ADHD. This is counterproductive. When you provide an explanation, there needs to be a solution. Often, one of the solutions for ADHD is medication. Why? So, we can help the child to conform to the behaviours that we want.

How backward is that? Now, I am not saying to not use medications. Nor am I saying that every child with ADHD actually has a compromised learning profile.

What I am saying is that we need to listen to what is happening for the child, within the child, to empower the child to be their best self. This is what precedes desirable behaviour. This is what feeds motivation to succeed.

What I am suggesting is that when we understand the behaviour as communication, we can target the underlying cause. This leads to desirable behaviours. Some children with ADHD received a diagnosis when the underlying cause is that they *learn* differently. The stress of navigating this difference lends to the symptoms of ADHD.

We need to look at the effect of the environment on the child, instead of the effect of the child's behaviour on the environment.

I worked with a seven-year-old school girl that was being treated for anger issues, impulsivity, and a pending ADHD or Oppositional Defiance Disorder diagnosis. She had exploded in a classroom, yelling and screaming as she overturned desks in the classroom. Her classmates had to be relocated for their safety.

This seven-year-old became a safety concern for the school. I am not sure about you, but I can't remember the last time I was concerned for my safety because of a seven-year-old!

What was the underlying cause of this lovely young girl's behaviour? She had been a target for her fellow classmates. New to the school, this client was incredibly hurt by the active exclusion by her classmates. This was a religious school of a minority group, where inclusion was an expected part of the community.

The day of the incident was caught on camera to provide evidence for the parents of how *out of control* their child was. This young girl had gone to the teacher for help and the situation was dismissed by the teacher.

Fear had been building over time. In this moment, the child was told that she was on her own. Her survival system went to work to protect her, because no one else would.

That is how you get a seven-year-old to exhibit behaviours that scare adults. You deny them protection, sparking their protection brain, the Emotional Brain, to take over. The body floods with adrenaline to provide enough strength energy to keep the child safe. Her message became BIGGER, LOUDER, STRONGER.

Do you think someone finally listened?!

After a few weeks of building rapport, the one thing that helped this child the most was one of the last days we worked together. We filled the room with about 17 balloons and allowed her to feel her anger as she popped the balloons with a pen.

We unleashed the anger on the teacher, on the students, and anything else that came to mind. Her parents reported that she was different after. She was calmer, laughing, and engaging again. Her fear of going anywhere without mom was melting away. All she needed was to be heard!

Again, we need to look at the effect of the environment on the child, instead of the effect of the child's behaviour on the environment.

Then, you can help support the weakness through understanding the child. By building upon the strengths, rather than changing the way they behave. When your child feels understood, she will take care of that on her own. When your child feels understood, there will be less symptomatic behaviour.

Your child is trying to do the best she can with the resources she has. She needs you to be patient and to be her guide through this growing up process.

When you *listen* to what the behaviour is communicating, your child will grow. You have the opportunity to understand, to nurture, and to guide your child. This helps your child to connect to herself. This self-connection is the best motivator for desirable behaviours.

What is driving your child's behaviour is not going to go away with teaching and coaching. When your child believes that something is wrong with who they are as a person, they will act out. Somewhere deep inside your child, she believes that she is worth more than that.

The behaviour is a desperate plea for a caring adult that can set boundaries. Her acting out is a plea for someone to care enough to be there. A loving adult with the strength to stay neutral or solid when she is emotional. This strength is what nurtures her ability to manage her emotions. A child that can manage her emotions is a child that is connected to herself. You are what your child needs to grow.

When you *listen*, you *hear* their soul! When your child feels heard, the most magical experience takes place. This is the key to your child feeling like an important, strong, powerful force of nature. This is the force of nature that drives an individual to be the best they can be.

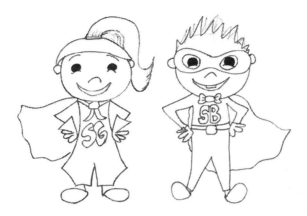

Your child wants to be the best version of himself and needs you to help him get there.

But, what if your child is over-reactive?

There is no such thing as overreaction. Your child *reacts* as his brain sees fit. If you think it's overreacting it means that the emotion is too great for you. You are the one that needs to do something about that. Not your child.

Your child is not responsible for your emotions.

In your child's mind, his reaction is exactly what is necessary. His brain works to take care of him. It does not choose to react based on what you may think is best for the situation. Your child's mind drives the behaviour whether you think it is a good decision or not.

So, how do you handle a child with questionable behaviour? You *grow* the child. Sam did not need to *learn* how to behave better. What Sam needed was to *experience* an interaction that *cultivates* self-regulation. In turn, this leads to better behaviour because he wants to be the best version of himself. He wants to succeed.

That's why he wanted to play in the first place. He thought that he was good enough. He wanted to get better. He instinctively knew that playing with the bigger boys would improve his skills and would show that he was capable.

When you help your child to manage his emotions, the Thinking Brain goes to work growing your child. With support, your child reflects on the situation and problem solves in a way that alters subsequent encounters with rejection. Next time, he will manage himself better because this was *cultivated within him*, not because it was taught to him.

You cultivate emotion regulation when you listen to what is happening within your child. When you identify the emotion that your child is feeling. When you validate what your child is experiencing and when you connect with his experience. I call this LIVE, and we will go over this in more detail in Chapter 11.

CHAPTER 7:
The Physiology of Emotion

"As soon as I saw you, I knew an adventure was going to happen."
- WINNIE-THE-POOH

In chapter 5, we talked about the *experience* of emotion. Now let's talk about the effect of emotion.

Imagine a bucket full of smooth, calm water.

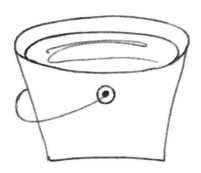

Imagine you toss a pebble into the bucket of water and small ripples form.

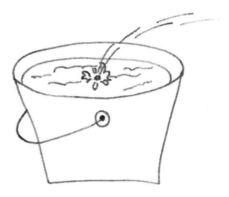

Imagine you toss a rock into the bucket and larger ripples form.

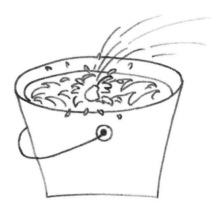

Imagine you wait. Eventually, the water returns to smooth calmness.

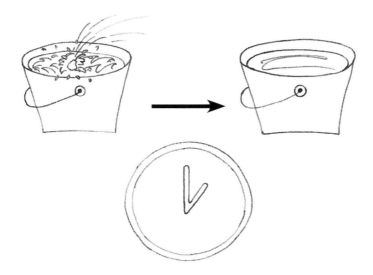

Imagine you are the bucket and your child is the water.

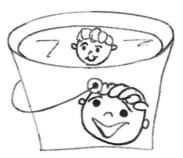

The pebbles and rocks are stressors in your child's life. Stress can be family, peers, school, activities, etc. Stress is the energy created by the body to help your child to get through the experience. The ripples in the water represent the emotional energy that your child feels in these situations.

As the bucket, you can feel the energy coming from the ripples in the water. But you must remain firm. As the bucket, you have to *hold the space* for your child.

When you *hold the space,* you do not absorb your child's energy. Absorbing your child's energy will affect your own energy. This can make you emotional. This can make you feel out of control. This can make you say or do things that only make the situation more intense.

Your intention is to make the situation change. You want your child to stop doing that, saying that, making that noise, or whatever else it may be. But when you react to what your child is doing, you are full of their energy as well as your own. You have become a flimsy bucket that is moved by the rippling water.

You have absorbed your child's energy and added it to your own. When you react to your child you put more energy into the situation. The edges of your flimsy bucket transfer energy back into the water and increase the amount of time until the water can calm.

For example, when your child throws a fit because you put limits on their screen-time, you can not engage in the battle. When you become defensive, YOU ARE AFFECTED. When you react, YOU ARE ENGAGED. Your child's energy is wanting to get you affected. This gives them power to make change. The change they want is to fulfill their 'need'.

This is not a conscious decision for your child. They are programmed to push boundaries. They are programmed to grow and expand.

56

What your child actually needs is for you to place healthy boundaries. And, you have to be immovable. You would simply reiterate the rules and not engage in an argument. You do not have to entertain all the comments about being a terrible parent and hearing how ALL the other children get freedoms that they do not.

It's like growing roses. If you let a rose bush grow wild, the bush will produce flowers. If you prune and care for the bush along the way, you produce a plant full of beautiful flowers.

To help your child grow, you must be immovable. The firmer your bucket, the stronger the child. This does not mean that you won't feel your child's emotions. Nor does it mean that you won't be affected by your child's emotions.

What it does mean is that your child's emotions cannot hijack your own.

Remember: the Emotional Brain is non-verbal and irrational. You are not helping the situation when you respond with emotion. You're just saying that taking care of you is more important than taking care of your child. And in turn, you reveal that you don't know how to take care of you.

Feeling comfortable with your own emotions means that your child's emotion cannot take over. When you engage with your child's energy, it increases the emotion of the moment. Unfortunately, what tends to happen is that we blame our children for our intense reaction.

Instead, allow your child the space to swash back and forth while you remain unmovable. Don't be afraid of her energy. *Hold the space* until she is able to settle back into calmness. When you do this, her emotional system re-corrects; it adjusts itself to act in a different way the next time around.

Your child's emotional system wants to be managed. This is the root of maturation. Maturity is when you can manage your emotions. Your child cultivates the ability to manage her emotions when you remain still.

You must be the solid that holds your child together. Even when you feel like you're going to wash away yourself, someone else needs to be your bucket. It cannot be your child.

You can sense the energy produced by the emotions of your child. The tantrum, the loud voice, slamming doors, stomping feet. It threatens your own system. It's tempting to take on this energy.

Your child's emotions can feel very uncomfortable. This is why it feels uncomfortable for you. Her system screams for help and you feel like you have to respond. You're the boss. You want to tell your child what to do, to demand certain behaviour, to provide consequences. But, is that effective? Usually not!

We can use the average garden ant to illustrate this concept.

When you step on an ant, the ant sends out a signal that communicates danger to the surrounding ants. The ants scurry, reinforcing this message.

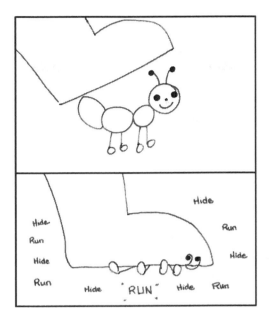

When you react to your child's emotions, the energy that over-powers them overpowers you. Your child experiences that their world is not safe. They feel insignificant as you are not there to protect them. You cannot withstand their powerful energy. You are both in danger.

Unless your child is in immediate danger, there is no need to get pulled into this energy.

You get pulled into this energy to help your child, but also to rid yourself of discomfort. You don't like that feeling that comes from your child's unbridled emotion. Your reaction is to take care of you.

You need to take care of both of you. You need to be the firm bucket for your child's moving energy. In the face of dysregulation, your child needs your strength to regain peace. This way, you both feel strong, safe, and significant. When you *hold the space*, you both grow.

You must not become reactive when your child is emotional. This is too much for your child to bear. This will teach your child to be...emotional!

The good news is that you don't have to be great at this yourself. You can work on managing your emotions at the same time. You have an advantage over your child. You are older and wiser. We think this means that we can 'teach' our children. But what it really means is that you can use it to grow you. *Then* your child will grow.

Emotional well-being comes when you and your child can regulate together. When you do not get pulled into your child's energy, you provide a space where their energy can re-correct. The purpose of emotion is to communicate. So, let it communicate.

Just Listen!

The Emotional Brain will settle, and the Thinking Brain will get to work. Your child's Thinking Brain is desperate to get to work. It wants to become the amazing person that is deep inside.

CHAPTER 8:

The Purpose of Emotion.

"When life throws you a rainy day, play in the puddles."
- WINNIE-THE-POOH

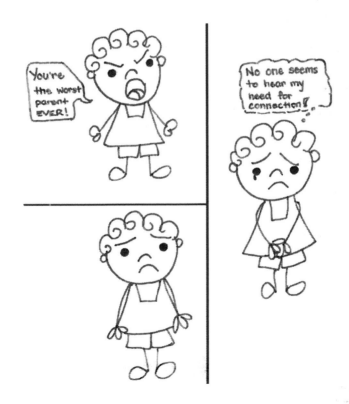

The purpose of emotion is to communicate. Emotion communicates what is going on inside your child. Your response to this communication impacts your child's emotional well-being. The more you listen, the better the outcome.

Listening is more than hearing with your ears. Listening is tuning in to the cues that your child's body is providing. Listening is attunement to the energy that is forming inside your child. Energy that is looking for a release.

To attune to your child is one of your most powerful assets as a parent. Your attentiveness can give you the power to hear what your child is communicating. And, when you know what is being communicated, you have the power to influence. How you respond is paramount.

Listening also includes attunement to the energy that comes from within yourself. When you are in tune, you understand that your body is communicating. What is being communicated is your own body's response to a situation.

When tensions rise within you, the natural inclination is to react. This happens when your child is not getting ready fast enough in the morning. This happens when it's the fifth time that you have asked your child to complete a task. You want to use a bit more force in your voice or in your words to motivate your child to action.

How you respond is the most crucial moment of helping your child to manage their emotions. You want this, because emotional regulation is the root of individual strength.

When tensions rise, it is the result of your child's emotional energy, plus your own. Your reaction can make matters worse.

This is much like the classic science experiment of the exploding volcano. Imagine that your child's emotion is the baking soda inside the volcano plug. Your emotional state is the vinegar. When you pour the vinegar into the baking soda, you get an explosive response.

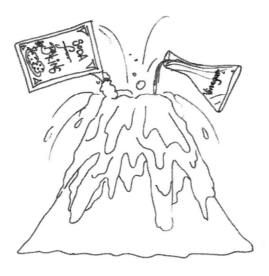

Baking Soda (*child's emotion*) + Vinegar (*parent's emotion*) = Explosion.

If you don't want an explosion, don't pour the vinegar onto the baking soda!

When we become emotional, we increase the chance of an explosion.

Your intention is to manage your child's emotional state. But instead, the situation gets worse. Everyone is more emotional. Your child is feeling like something is wrong with him. He is feeling scared.

You may excuse this behaviour thinking you need to teach your child. You're the boss! But excuses don't raise children. Unfortunately, they have the power to create the feelings of shame and internalized hatred for oneself. But don't worry. Children are resilient and highly receptive to parents that are always trying to improve.

The result is a child that feels defective, especially if your verbal language is hurtful. Your emotional response is penetrating. Your child thinks that something is wrong with *him*. He feels shame, guilt, even fear.

This was not your intention. You felt your own surge of discomfort. But, you took care of your feelings instead of your child's. You didn't mean to do it that way. But that is what it means for your child.

The *intention* of your emotion was to communicate to your child that you were not pleased with him. The *purpose* of your emotion was to create change. Something *was* wrong. It could have been his behaviour or his actions that needed to change. As the parent, you stepped in. Makes sense, but this is not how your child will see things.

Your child will integrate that *he* is the problem, not his *behaviour*, but him the *person*. Your child does not have the capacity to separate his value from his behaviour.

Children that think they are a problem become self-fulfilling prophecies. They become *problem* children because they *learn* who they are *through* you. How you interact with your child teaches them *who* they are.

Your child connects to you when you can manage your emotions. Your child connects to himself when he can manage his emotions (especially with your support). We all want to be connected.

If you have a hard-enough time managing your own emotions, how can you expect your child to do so?

Your emotion is there to warn you and to protect you. Emotion is real. It is neither good nor bad. How we act on the emotion can become a problem. When a child's emotional state is threatening to disrupt our own, this is not an invitation to act on your emotions.

This can lead to reprimanding, ignoring or minimizing your child, which is hurtful, for both of you. What is beneficial to both of you is your ability to not engage with their dysregulation. There is another way to support your child through this process.

You need to manage your emotions for your child to learn that they have value. This is how you cultivate emotional well-being. When your child's emotion threatens your internal state, you first need to tend to you. You need to contain your emotions. You need to refrain from interactions with your child until you can remain *neutral*.

Neutral is the state where you are the firm, immovable bucket that holds the space. This is the space where your child's emotions can work their way out. This is the space where you and your child grow together. This is where connections form, connections to oneself and connections to others.

Building connection is another purpose of emotion. We connect to ourselves when we can tolerate the discomforts that well up within us. We connect to others when we can tolerate the discomforts that exist in their presence. The best listeners are those that can hear others' emotions yet remain neutral. Listening shows that we care, while remaining strong enough to not get pulled in. This is the source of connection.

Don't worry! If you fear you have already messed up, you probably have. You **will** mess up. That's why it's not just what you do that matters.

It's what you do after what you've done.

Apologize to your child when you mess up. Take ownership, explain what you did wrong and how you will work to improve. Work on improving together. This makes for beautiful bonding on a level that feels amazing!!

PART C:
THE BOUNDARY

How often do you hear someone say, *you just need to love yourself?* There is a popular '80's song that claims that it is the greatest gift of all. But really, what does it mean to *love yourself?*

What if a more accurate phrase was *be content* with yourself. And to be *content* with yourself was to feel connected in a way were nothing could shake you. Where you would feel firm in your space. Where you would feel comfortable simply being with you.

This is the essence of a boundary. The ability to know what space is yours and what space is not yours. What you are responsible for, and what you are not responsible for. That you no longer have to carry the weight of emotions and behaviours that don't belong to you.

I believe that this is at the core of knowing yourself. That loving yourself is actually a plea to be connected with yourself.

You have to be connected to yourself before you can connect to another. The problem we have is that we try to use others to feel connected without first being connected to our self.

Your child's behaviour is most likely a plea to feel connected, to feel like they belong. The most powerful way for you to give this *gift* to your child, is for you to be connected to yourself, and to help her connect to herself.

This is done through healthy boundary setting. This section will walk you through how to use boundaries to grow both of you. Growth in a love for the self and a love for each other.

CHAPTER 9:

Separateness

*"We didn't realize we were making memories.
We just knew we were having fun!"*
- WINNIE-THE-POOH

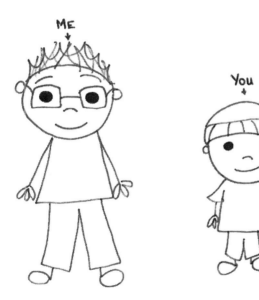

Understanding separateness is important in your child's development as an individual. When it comes to humans, a boundary is the division between what is yours and what is mine. It is what separates you from me.

Separateness is knowing that your emotions belong to you and your child's emotions belong to them. You are not responsible for your child's emotions. You are responsible for how you interact with her emotions, but you are not responsible for how she *experiences* her emotion.

When you feel responsible for your child's emotions, you may think it's an invitation to *control* the emotion. For example, "Stop that right now!", "You're OK!", "You're overreacting!". Your child's *out-of-control* energy will be inviting you to come and *control* her.

You must resist this seemingly desperate plea as it undermines the process of growing up confident. No one can *control* another person's emotions. You cannot *control* what your child feels inside.

What you can do is influence your child's *experience* with the emotion. When you set a boundary, you say, "That is yours and this is mine." Which actually says, "I can't take care of that feeling *for* you. But what I can do is *be right here for you* while you go through it. It may be uncomfortable, but you will make it through. I love you. I am right here!"

The only way for your child to manage their emotions is to go through it. She must go into it. "Feel the force Luke!" for all you Star Wars fans. To feel it and to tolerate it is how we grow.

It's like physically training the body. The more you go into the pain, the stronger you will become. The only difference here is that you are building your child's emotional self, instead of her physical self.

Nurturing your child's emotional self is how she grows closer to you. And, how she grows closer to herself. When she feels in touch with herself, she feels powerful. Once connected to herself, she is motivated to become the amazing force that is inside of her.

Your child's greatest challenge in life will be to manage her own force of nature. Your child's greatest strength in life will be the management of her emotions.

Your child will find success in anything they do when they take responsibility for what is theirs. Success will be when your child can own their emotions and have the power to face them.

You set your child up for success when you nurture the ability to tolerate discomfort. To meet the emotion head on. When your child knows that you won't *take on* their emotions, but you will be *right there* while they work through it. Your child needs your strength to become a strength of their own.

This is how you get your child's emotion to calm. This is the way to restore harmony in the body and let the Thinking Brain get back to work towards growth. This is the way to master the self.

Your relationship with your child is one of their most valuable resources. Unhealthy relationships confuse the line between what is yours and what is mine. Unhealthy relationships include making other people responsible for your emotions.

We need to stay away from this. Parents often perpetuate a toxic environment and then place blame on their children. Parents blame children when they react with anger or frustration.

Healthy relationships can separate the difference and be okay with that.

You are responsible for your emotions. Your child is responsible for theirs. How you feel in a situation is your own *experience*. How you behave is *your* responsibility. Your child may be the kindling, but they are not *responsible* for your emotions. You are!

When your child creates an emotional response within you, your child is not the source of your upset. The source is the discomfort that you feel at the expense of the stimuli coming from your child. What you are feeling has to do with all the stored-up garbage that you carry.

So, you can't blame your child when you react to her emotion. You are responsible not to react. You are responsible to have firm boundaries in place. The boundaries that separate you from me. What is mine and what is yours.

How you respond will set the tone of your relationship with your child. This directly influences how your child handles her own emotions and how your child feels about herself.

You must tend to your own discomfort. You need to heal whatever is driving your own pain. Commit to your own resolve and keep this energy from your child. The discomfort is yours, not theirs.

You are your child's mentor. Your child relies on you to set the tone for how to interact with her emotions. Keeping the two of you separate grows both of you at the same time. When you manage your emotions, your child feels safe and supported. When you don't engage with her emotions, you communicate that you can manage her overpowering sensations. This gives her strength. She will follow your lead.

If you want your child to be calmer, happier, and more regulated, you first have to model how to do this. It is important to note that regulating emotions is not the same as hiding emotion. Ignoring or suppressing your own emotions is counterproductive. It is like pushing a beach ball under the water until it bops you in the face.

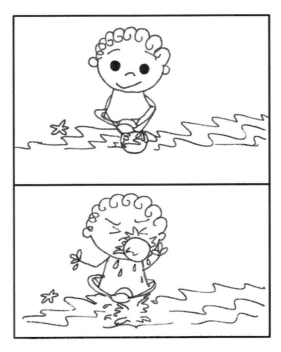

Ignoring emotion is not the same as being neutral. Neutral is listening to yourself and tending to your needs without engaging. Then, allowing space for your child to work through her stuff.

Strength and stillness come from your ability to tend to your own emotional space. You take a moment when you need to. You interact when you can remain neutral.

A boundary ensures that your emotions remain yours, and your child's emotions remain your child's.

When your child is emotional, you don't take this on either.

When your moody teenager tries to engage you in her sullenness, you do not match her behaviour. Nor, do you mock and tease. When your toddler starts to scream for more cookies, you do not entertain a rationale. Nor, do you start yelling at your little one.

The purpose of the boundary is to provide space for growth and maturation for your child. You acknowledge your child's emotional state. You help them to meet the emotion. You guide your child in listening to her emotions. To understand herself and not be afraid. You keep what is yours, and you help her through what is hers.

Each child is like a tree. Self-regulation is the roots of a tree. A storm is the stressors of life. The deeper the roots reach into the ground, the less likely the tree is to be uprooted in a storm.

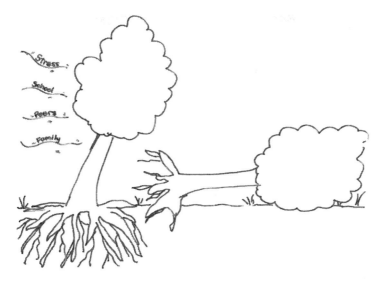

The roots grow deeper every time there is an emotional storm, and you do not get pulled in. You are there to support your child, but you do not engage in the emotion. When the storm comes, you safely hold your place in the storm because of the depth of your own roots.

The healthy boundaries you place will grow the roots of her tree. If your roots are not very deep, then you need to start growing your own. Your child cannot do this for you. You will have to find a strong adult to do this. You are your own tree. Your child is her own tree. Your support is essential for her to grow her roots of emotional regulation.

LISTEN!

CHAPTER 10:

Togetherness

"If there ever comes a day when we can't be together, keep me in your heart and I will be there forever!"
- CHRISTOPHER ROBIN

In your child's journey to become separate, he cannot do it alone. Research shows that the greatest detriment to a child's development is abuse and neglect. We need connectedness to grow.

Your child needs connection to thrive. The primary caregiver is the first point of contact for emotional regulation. Your child was born raw and unable to manage his own emotions. It is in the presence of others that he develops this skill.

How you react or respond to your child is paramount. When you meet your child's needs, he is calm. When your child's needs are not met, he is uncomfortable. His reaction is an unbridled call for help.

For example, after a long day, your child wants to have some extra screen-time. He was up early in the morning for run club. He then made it through another self-proclaimed boring day of school. After school he went to basketball practice and suffered through an undesirable dinner selection.

You're not surprised as he begins a debate about your rules.

You are very tired yourself and the last thing you want to do is to deal with another emotional upheaval. Faster than you can think, *"No!"* leaves your mouth and a bellowing cry shrieks through the house.

Your beloved child has turned into a bundle of evil. You hear obscenities from your child's mouth. And then he screams his most powerful weapon, "You're the worst parent in the world. I hate you!"

In this moment, you have one of three options (and no, shipping your child off to boarding school is not one of them)!

Option #1

Ignore your child and walk away.

You have had a long day. You cannot tolerate one more outburst from your child. You don't want to be a part of this. You need to be far away, and you take your leave.

The Result:

He gets louder and the behaviour becomes more intense. When you ignore the Emotional Brain, it says, "I guess you can't hear me!" So, it gets BIGGER, LOUDER and STRONGER.

It is one of the most powerful parts of you. The Emotional Brain KEEPS YOU ALIVE! If the Emotional Brain thinks that you are not listening, it will do EVERYTHING to make itself heard. Even if that means eating your child up inside without you even knowing about it.

So, your child internalizes that his world is not safe. His energy was too much for you. It was powerful enough to make you walk away. But you're supposed to be his protection. You left him. You abandoned him when he needed you.

He begins to sense that something is wrong with him. The emotion that was too much for him is too much for you. He feels out of control and no one is there to be his safety. No one is there to be his bucket. Your child develops the sense that he is defective and fears that there is no one that can 'handle' him.

Option #2

Engage with your child by matching his behaviour.

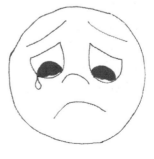

This emotion is too much for you. You feel agitated. You raise your voice and demand that your child stop the behaviour. You threaten what will happen if they do not stop.

The Result:

You basically became the same age as your child. You matched his energy, which is driven by fear. For your child, he was presenting a need. It may not have been a need, but your child believes that it is.

Your engagement with the uncomfortable emotion magnified its energy. You became the same age as your child. You communicated that you could be overcome by the energy, so you are weak.

The makes your child feel scared. He internalizes that his world is not safe. His energy was powerful enough to activate you and make *you* defensive and scared.

You are his mentor and you are nurturing insecurity and fear. He begins to develop shame and guilt, as he feels responsible for your behaviour.

Option #3:

Stay with your child and set healthy boundaries.

You listen to what your child's behaviour is communicating. You identify the emotion. You validate the reason for her response. You empathize with your child.

These four steps are the basis of LIVE, a step-by-step process that we will discuss in Chapter 11 to assist you in cultivating emotional regulation in your child.

The Result:

Your child feels your presence. He senses your boundary which helps him to recorrect his energy. You do not take on his emotions, so you do not add to the discomfort that he is already experiencing. His emotions remain in his own space.

He sees that you can tolerate his emotions. You model strength. He draws on this strength to not be afraid of the discomfort that he feels inside. He tolerates his own emotions. His emotions begin to settle. He feels connected to you. He feels connected to himself.

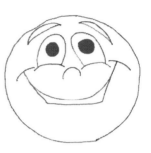

In the third option, you guide your child through the process of tolerance. You help your child to work through the energy that is mounting in his body. He learns how to be okay with feeling uncomfortable. He learns that this will pass and on the other side is peace, clarity, and safety.

When your child is upset, he feels something inside himself. There is an intense energy surging through his body. The energy is created by the body to make something happen. The energy is overwhelming, confusing, even frightening. The energy needs to go somewhere. It usually comes out in challenging behaviours.

Reprimand, punishment, or blame adds to the overwhelming experience. Your child's behaviour is calling for help. When your child receives rejection, it hurts.

What your child needs is compassion. He needs you to *listen*. He needs you to *hold the space*, not to punish or walk away when he is out-of-control.

You must be the bucket that holds the space for your child until his system can calm. Until he feels settled. You, the adult, become the temporary boundary while your child gradually develops a boundary of his own.

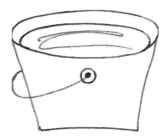

Every time you experience option number three, your child's boundary system strengthens. If you are thinking that this is not an easy task, YOU'RE SO RIGHT!

Children push your boundaries to grow. Remember Mowgli from Chapter One? Your child needs to explore to learn about her environment. Expect your child to push, test, and to challenge your boundary system. Plan on it!

Each time you give in, your child's boundary system weakens. Resorting to option one or option two fosters pain, insecurity, and weakness. When your child can push your boundaries, the attention turns to meeting *your* needs, not your child's.

This is a natural response! Your Emotional Brain will turn on for your own preservation. You react on your emotion. It may stop the behaviour in the short term. In the long run, it hurts both of you.

What you do in this moment is about control and the need to change the situation. If you want to teach your child that power is the boss, he will learn that fear is more important than strength.

When you react to your child, you are modelling that their emotions are more powerful than you. This communicates weakness and insecurity. Whatever your child did to cause you to get activated is due to your own stuff. Contain your emotions and channel your discomfort away from your child. Help ease your child's discomfort by holding the space.

Matt, an international business owner, wanted help in growing his 11-year-old's self-esteem. Matt suspected that his anger issues may have something to do with Jack's low self-image.

Matt and I worked together to identify his triggers. As is often the case, Jack had unresolved emotions related to baggage from his past. We went to work to heal the negative energies stored in his nervous system (using appropriate therapeutic interventions), and to recorrect the behaviours that hurt his relationship with his son.

I taught Matt the steps of LIVE and he put them to action!

This was the plan. When Matt felt angered by Jack, he excused himself for a moment and went to his man cave. Here, Matt expressed all the superlatives that flooded his mind. Then, Matt returned upstairs where he would join in a calm interaction with his son.

As was expected, upon his return, Jack would push, poke and prod Matt's every button, trying to get a response. But Matt did not allow himself to get pulled into Jack's emotion.

The result was a powerful, non-verbal communication. What was communicated through Dad's actions was that Dad is strong. Dad is strong because he can manage the powerful force of emotion that wells within himself. Dad is strong because he is not swayed by his child's powerful energy.

This is when a child grows. Your child cannot grow without you. This is the space where your child grows closer to himself and closer to you.

You must be the solid in their fluid world. You must be the bucket. When you establish firm boundaries, you do not give them what is yours. Your child learns what is theirs and they become responsible for that, because you nurtured this. You cultivated this. They grow in the management of their emotions, which is the root and foundation of growing a strong self.

CHAPTER 11:
How to *Hold the Space*

"It makes such a difference to have someone who believes in you!"
- WINNIE-THE-POOH

The most effective way to nurture your child's emotional well-being is to *hold the space*. Every time you're immovable in the face of your child's unbridled emotion, your child gains strength. Every time your child disrupts your own stability, you both weaken.

Your child is the greatest threat to your own emotional well-being. Your child is a part of you. You have invested mentally, emotionally, physically, and financially in raising this individual. She is a reflection of you.

Your child stimulates strong emotions inside of you. Your emotions play a role because of your connection and your investment. If you cannot manage your own emotions, your child will not be able to manage hers. There is no way around that.

I have come up with an acronym to guide you through the steps of cultivating emotional regulation in your child. To help your child manage her emotions, use LIVE.

Listen
Identify
Validate
Empathize

Listen

Listening is more than what you do with your ears. Listening to your child is more than hearing the words they speak. Listening includes observing what her body is communicating. You need to listen to hear the message the emotion is conveying.

Generally, behaviour is the first indicator that your child is activated. When your child is affected, step back from the situation. Take note of what is going on. Be a detective.

The behaviour is a symptom of what is happening inside your child.

Listen to yourself. Take note of how you are feeling inside. Do you feel a strong emotion coming on? Do you want to act quickly to change what is happening? Can you keep your cool?

Do not *REACT* to the behaviour. Reacting includes any emotional response by you. You can tell if your response is emotional if you get defensive, upset, agitated, or impatient. You are now activated, and your emotional energy rises. This energy is going to want to do something. How you manage this energy contributes to your child's emotional success.

Reacting is when you only focus on the behaviour. Targeting the behaviour alone misses out on a very important step in learning how to manage emotions. Yes, the behaviour may be unacceptable or concerning. But, if the behaviour becomes the focus, you are not hearing the message.

Think of a time when a boss, family member, or partner focused on your *behaviour* and not your situation. Did you feel understood and supported, or did you feel defensive and misunderstood?

The situation is no different for your child. Your child is doing her best. She needs your help through this moment, not your disregard. Use her behaviour for cues that can explain what might be happening for her.

Listen to understand your experience in the moment. Listen to understand your child's experience in the moment.

Identify

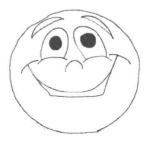

Once you listen to your child's experience, identify the emotions she is feeling.

Say, "You feel *sad!*", "You're *angry.*"

You're probably used to asking "What are your feelings? What is going on with you?"

Your child does not know the answer to this question.

Remember, the Emotional Brain is non-verbal. Your child's mind is limited in putting words to emotions. So, you will get the answer that you're seeking. Your child is programmed to mirror you. She will give you the answer that she thinks you want to hear.

How good are you at describing how or what you are feeling? How can you expect this of your child?

If you by-pass this step and go right to trying to manage the behaviour, the Emotional Brain gets grumpy. It says, "Hey, I guess you didn't hear me. I have a job to protect you. Since you missed my first message, I will send you another message that is *bigger, louder and stronger.*"

Your child's emotion intensifies!

If you react to your child's emotions, you add her energy to your own. This magnified emotion is directed at your child.

Your child's emotions intensify!!

She feels out of control. All your effort goes into making her stop because you feel out of control yourself.

To regain composure, first tend to your own emotional state. Step back emotionally. Take a moment. Do anything that interrupts your desire to react. It is okay to say you need a moment. But always add, "I'll be back shortly." to avoid feelings of abandonment or rejection. When you are ready, identify the emotion. Stay with the emotion.

This does not mean that you support the reactions of your child or condone her behaviour. Instead, you are cultivating self-regulation. The Emotional Brain does not care if you agree or not with what is happening. It requires acknowledgement to begin to deactivate, to shut itself off.

When you stay neutral with the emotion, you communicate that you are not intimidated. You are okay with what is happening inside of her. You are not judging her. You are *being with* her.

When you ask your child how she feels, her Emotional Brain becomes more activated. You're the person who's supposed to help her through this, so *you* should know the answer. Or at least, you should be working together to sort this out.

It's *your* job to tell your child what she's experiencing. You have to help her develop an understanding of herself. You are there to nurture an awareness of herself. She does not instinctively know how to do this. She instinctively knows how to need you. She needs you to cultivate the understanding by identifying what it is she is *experiencing*. To put into words what she is *feeling*.

You must point this out. Even if you are wrong, your child will correct you. Even if you are right, she may correct you! The important point is that you are working on this together.

What is crucial is that you identify the emotion. Because when you do this, the Emotional Brain feels satisfied and can begin to retreat. When you acknowledge the emotion, the Emotional Brain de-activates.

The Emotional Brain has a job to do. It keeps you alive. It does this by protecting you from threat. Any emotion felt by your child comes from her body's need to *do* something. The *something* always relates to survival.

This does not mean impending doom. Your child's needs include belonging, food, shelter, autonomy, competence and eventually, independence. It could be for social connection, to prove ability, or to meet basic bodily functions. Either way, your child's emotion is about the preservation of her!

The Emotional Brain knows that it has done its job when you acknowledge that it has spoken. When you do not listen, it will increase in intensity. When you *hear* it and *acknowledge* it, it will begin to settle down, to turn off.

Using phrases such as, "*You feel sad,*" "*You feel angry,*" "*You feel embarrassed,*" tell the Emotional Brain, I *HEAR* you. I *HEAR* the message that you are communicating.

This is how you get your child to begin to settle. This pushes the reset button on your child. The calming chemistry is released, the Thinking Brain starts to *come back* online, your child starts to come back to earth!

You may also need to remove the source of the stimuli. Being a detective can help you identify triggering context. The affective stimuli could be school, crowds, sounds, hunger, or exhaustion. You want to identify and remove the stimulus to the best of your ability. When this is not possible, focus on LIVE and build strength through awareness.

This is how your child learns to be with herself. You are modelling how to be okay when feeling intense emotion. You are guiding your child to connect with herself. Connecting to herself and being comfortable in her own emotion is the source of self-regulation. It is her source of peace.

Validate

Express understanding of the situation. State that you understand (or you are trying to) why your child responded the way she did.

"You are angry because _____."
"You are sad because_____."

This shows that you get it! When you show that you *get it*, it lessens the power of the emotion. You *heard* what was communicated, so there is no need to communicate further.

Empathize

"I'd be upset too if my friends didn't invite me to the party!"

Show that it makes sense. Show that the behaviour, in context, makes sense. Again, this does not mean that you agree with the behaviour. What is does say is that you are trying to understand why your child became so reactive.

This is such a powerful moment for your child. This is the most powerful way to grow strength in your child.

Emotion is neither good nor bad. It just is. What we do with emotion can be considered good or bad, but emotion alone is simply an experience within the self.

The experience of emotion can be overwhelming. When you react negatively to your child's emotions, she learns that she is a problem. When you help her through the emotional experience, she learns that she is pricelessly invaluable and important. Her importance comes from a solid feeling of connection to herself because she can tolerate the powerful energy that is she.

The Result

When you follow these steps, your child's mind will start to calm down. Her demeanor will start to settle. Her problem-solving Thinking Brain will start to work once again.

When you help your child through the emotion process, they regain composure. They have clear and rational thought. This is when teaching can be effective.

But hang on! Before sharing your parental wisdom, check in to see what your child can contribute. Once your child regains composure, engage her mind in the problem-solving experience. Guide her through the *thinking* process.

Use the questions that come into your mind to help your child generate her own thoughts and solutions about the situation!

Ask,

What happened?

What would you like to have happen?

What could you do differently next time?

What could I do differently next time?

Her mind will assimilate new information, including lessons learned about her discomfort. When you *hold the space* for your child, her mind will be less reactive. The next time a situation occurs, she will be less intense because her mind has adapted.

You can fill in the gaps with your own wisdom along the way. But first, lead your child's mind to do the work. You will set your child up for success in the world where emotions are at play every single day.

Your child's mind craves learning. It wants to grow, to expand and to mature. Emotional moments are not setbacks, but opportunities to grow. Emotion is an invitation to understand your inner world. It is an invitation to understand your child's inner world. Your child will connect to herself through the management of her emotions.

Story Time

The following are three stories that illustrate the importance of holding the space.

School Refusal

The following is a conversation between a client and me.

Mom: Mia is refusing to go to school. I can't get her into the car. We missed the first few days because we were still on holiday and she is refusing to go. I'm going to be late for work and I'll get fired if this keeps happening!

Me: Oh dear.

Mom: Sorry to bother you but help! Please.

Me: Hear her words, see her body language, acknowledge the emotion, "Mia, I can see you are angry because we missed the first few days of school."

Mom: Okay, I'll try. (We had talked about this a lot, so this was more a reminder).

(elapsed time)

Mom: You'll never guess what happened. I told her how I knew she was scared because I could see how badly she didn't want to get in the car. Then I crouched down in the car and acted scared. I said that I know what it is like because I used to be scared of going to school. Then SHE GOT IN HER CAR SEAT AND SAID, "Let's go!" Thank you!

In this account, mom followed the steps of LIVE.

Mom **L**istened to her daughter's words and body language.
"Mia is refusing to get in the car."

Mom **I**dentified the emotion that Mia was feeling.
"I see you are angry/scared."

Mom **V**alidated the feeling by showing understanding for the source of the emotion.
"I know you're angry because we missed the first few days of school."

Mom **E**mpathized by showing understanding of the display of emotion.
"I used to be scared of going to school."

Using **LIVE** helped to deactivate the emotion. Then Mia's mind could come up with a solution instead of being in the emotional space.

Teen Using Marijuana

Concerned parents had contacted me because of the mounting stress in their home. Their eldest child, a 15-year-old son, was becoming increasingly distant and closed off. The parents were blaming the behaviour on their son's use of marijuana.

Every attempt to keep him close was unsuccessful. They had done the usual, including lecturing about the long-term harmful effects of drug use and their expectations for his behaviour.

The parents asked if I could get their son to stop using marijuana. I made it clear that there is nothing I can do to make that happen unless that was what their son wanted.

"Okay, then. Can you make him *want* to stop using?" was the parents' desperate alternate plea.

Again, my message was clear. As parents, they have more power than anyone to influence what their child chooses to do. I could work with the son on creating a connection which would then help with their own. More importantly, if they were to incorporate **LIVE**, they would see a shift in their son's world and in the life of their family.

Using **LIVE** helps your child to connect to you, and to connect to himself. Children want to please those with whom they have a connection. This is the underlying root to motivating your child to make good decisions. Help him connect to you by nurturing the connection to himself.

What was important for this family was the parents' efforts. They traded in ultimatums and contracts to reignite their connection with their son. They needed to shift their efforts from *lecturing* to *listening*. Lecturing is a tangible way to help a parent feel better. It is not effective in helping your child, unless you want to push your child away.

The parents implemented coaching tips on how to navigate the situation. First, they had to manage their conflict with each other. When parents argue, fight or feel feisty with a partner, children feel insecure and scared. A child may also feel responsible and take the blame when they cannot make it go away. This always affects a child's behaviour. The couple worked on not fighting in front of their son, especially when arguing about him.

I explained **LIVE** to the parents. I told them to forget about the substance use for the time being. The focus on this behaviour pushed their son away. I explained that the substance use was the symptom, not the problem. Substance use comes from dealing with internal pain.

To influence change in their son, they would need to reconnect. They would need to start *listening*.

Listen.

The parents acknowledged the substance use as a choice their son was making. They reiterated that they still did not agree with his drug use, but they were not going to try and make him stop. This communicated that they were open to hearing his heart.

A child is desperate to give their heart to someone who will listen. A child will not give their heart to someone who is judgmental or critical.

Identify.

The parents were unsure what their teenage son was feeling. According to the teenager, he was fine and not feeling anything. So, we went with what we knew, "You're angry because we are on your case to stop using weed." That was a given. Not the true source of any drive for drug use, but it worked for now. It showed an attempt to be understanding.

When you point out an emotion, you may experience resistance. Don't get pulled in. It's the effort that counts with this population. Identify what you notice in your teen. Refrain from analysis, judgement, or advice.

This is a delicate area when dealing with an adolescent. A teenager wears different masks daily. This stage in life is about finding out who you are. The teenage brain is raw and emotional.

Validate.

The parents expressed understanding that marijuana use was common with teens.

Empathize.

The parents acknowledged that it would be hard to stop, as marijuana use had been a habit for a long time. Also, the client was close to his uncle who had used for years and was "okay". And, it would be hard to quit if that was what his friends were doing.

The Result.

The son began to re-engage with the family. He appeared happier. He spent less time in his room and more time with his family. The parents' openness and willingness helped their son to feel valuable. Instead of feeling not valued, he felt warmth and belonging.

He felt happier at home. He was chattier and started to feel better about himself. The teen spoke about how difficult it was to quit because of the social and physiological factors. He was still using and that was not going to change anytime soon. But this is ultimately his decision. What was going to help in the long run was the connection he had to his parents and to himself.

In session, he went from a client that would sleep and hardly speak to being chatty and sharing personal information. The agenda was never to make him do or be what someone else wanted. The plan was always to help him to feel stronger from the inside out. This is how you empower your child to make good decisions.

We all need to feel a sense of belonging, especially the compromised emotional teenager. You cultivate a strong bond with your child through emotional mastery.

Lisa's Story

Lisa, a 14-year-old ninth grader, came up with an elaborate plan to gain favour with her peers. Unfortunately for Lisa, her plan went sideways. The experience would become a social embarrassment and an economic strain for the family.

I received a call from Lisa's mother, "What do I do? Dad has been out of town for work and is on his way home. I would rather tell him in person but if I don't call him, he may hear it from someone else. I don't want that to happen either."

What advice would you give?

"Decide if you want your husband to hear it from you by phone, or if you want to risk him finding out from another individual. But once he finds out, you must give him the following information!"

The following was my offer.

Dad had a choice. On the one hand, he could reprimand and lecture Lisa on all the things that she did wrong. He could add how this was going to negatively affect the family and how angry he was. What was she thinking?

The motivation to do this generally comes from a feeling that you need to do your due diligence as a parent. You need to provide a learning experience in the absence of good decision making.

What you don't realize is how your emotions can take over. Appeasing your own discomfort can become the primary goal, disguised as *teaching* your child.

The result is a child that shuts down. The child's mind feels attacked. Lisa's Emotional Brain will activate and her behaviour will be about survival.

In contrast, if Dad were to use **LIVE**, Lisa's brain will be accessible for learning, problem solving, and growth.

Dad was strong. Dad had wanted to come home and express his anger. He did not.

Listen.

He used a calm voice to acknowledge that they were all affected by the situation.

Identify.

Dad identified that *he* was angry and needed time to work through his own thoughts and feelings. He added that he had to take space to sort through his emotions instead of putting his anger on her. He acknowledged that this may be uncomfortable for her, but he will let her know when he would be ready to talk.

*V*alidate.

Dad expressed that he understood that the behaviour came from wanting to impress her peers.

Empathize.

Dad was able to say that he understood the need to fit in. He added that he knows that she did not plan for it to turn out the way that it did, and this was a harrowing experience for her as well.

Perfect!

If you've ever felt like giving your child the most profound lecture on poor decision making, this is how to do it. Without hardly saying anything at all. Simply and calmly say that you are disappointed. Your child's greatest hope is to make you happy and proud. Let your child's mind do the work.

Here is why.

When you lecture your child on what they did wrong, their mind switches to a state of defensiveness. Her Emotional Brain kicks in. In this state, your child will feel under threat. The Thinking Brain shuts off. The Emotional Brain kicks into gear to protect the child. You will lecture. They will not hear you.

When you are reactive and defensive, your child feels responsible. They feel like they are a *bad* person. Your child feels like she is bad, defective, a failure, a problem.

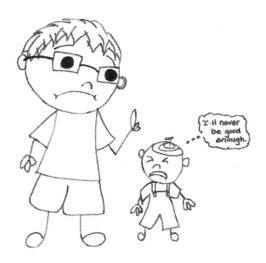

Your child's natural response is to reject this feeling. They may say, "I hate you. Get away from me. I want to run away. You don't care about me."

When you react with emotion, your child does not hear anything that you say. They feel your emotional upheaval. Your child *feels* everything that you say.

When you are angry, they *FEEL* that.

When you are scared, they *FEEL* that.

When you are sad, they *FEEL* that.

When you are embarrassed, the *FEEL* that.

When you are disgusted, they *FEEL* that.

When you are happy, they definitely *FEEL* that.

Not only does your child *FEEL* that, but she feels *responsible* for that.

Your child is not responsible for *your* emotion. You are responsible for your own self-regulation. You must tend to your charged emotion first.

If Lisa's parents were unable to manage their own emotions, Lisa would have felt that energy. She would have taken on their hurt, their anger, and their embarrassment. Lisa's mental efforts would have shifted to her own safety and survival, not to how to solve the problem.

Lisa's parents took the road less traveled. When the typical reaction would have been to punish extensively, they worked to *grow* their child through nurturance (and neuroscience!). There were many people that offered their input on how to handle the situation. These parents ignored the rumbles and turned their focus on growing their family.

The result for Lisa was that she displayed powerful and mature moments of growth. Her brain moved into a state of problem solving. She went to work to fix and repair all that she had done in a very impressive manner.

Help your child to have ownership of her own emotions. *Listen* to your child. She does not need your lectures. Her brilliant mind is waiting for you to set the stage for her growth. This is how your child learns. Nurture what is within her to be the teacher. Start the process by following **LIVE**.

When you hold the space for your child, she will grow in her ability to self-regulate. This leads to making the choices and decisions that drive mature behaviour.

CHAPTER 12:
The Result - A Happy Child.

"We will be friends forever, won't we Pooh?"
- PIGLET

"Even longer!"
- POOH

One of the greatest gifts you can give your child is a strong sense of self. You cannot teach this. You have to cultivate the ability to be okay with yourself.

A strong sense of self comes from knowing that you can trust yourself. Trusting yourself comes from knowing that you can face the stressors of life and survive. Trusting yourself comes from knowing that you can handle the emotional world and be okay.

Trust comes from a connection to the self. Our emotions have the power to disconnect us from ourself and from others. Emotions can be overwhelming and make us feel out of control. When we can be with our emotions and allow them to communicate, to do their job as they pass through, we grow stronger. The way to connect with yourself is in your capacity to self-regulate.

Emotions are like clouds full of rain. The clouds come in, squeeze out the water, and then move along and dissipate. Emotions are not meant to stick around and plague us. The more capable you are at tending to your emotions, the sooner they pass through.

Strong emotions are uncomfortable. Our mind wants to get rid of discomfort. We often attempt to get others to take this emotion from us so that we do not have to suffer. Yet, no one can take this emotion for you.

Your child cannot be the bearer of your emotion. A child is too fragile to be a bucket for an adult. You must be the bucket for your child. If you feel weak, your child will feel more fragile. You grow together as you work to strengthen yourself and become a firm bucket for your child. You grow in trusting yourself. You grow in connecting to yourself.

You also do not take on your child's emotions. You provide strength for your child. You make space for your child to experience and tolerate her own emotions. Your strength nurtures her strength. Her own self-regulation fosters strength.

The result,
  A grounded, happy, strong, capable child!

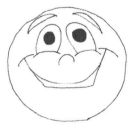

PART D:
AGE SPECIFIC
BEHAVIOUR

To grow a beautiful plant, you must meet its specific needs. The plant will require the correct balance of water, sunshine, and nutrient specific soil.

Growing a plant is like growing a child. Your child's job is to grow. He grows when his needs are met. Your job is to meet his needs, to the best of your ability.

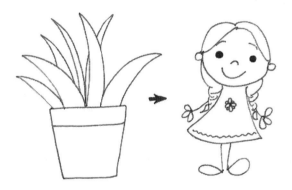

Your job is to provide the most optimal environment that you can. He needs you to provide the nutrient dense soil, the water, and the sunshine. When you provide these needs, your child thrives.

When a plant looks healthy, you feel good. When your child is doing well, you feel great.

When a plant is not looking so good, you wonder what went wrong. Was there too much water? Not enough water? I know this scenario far too well. I often think I am doing everything right, yet my plants rarely make it!

What I did not know is that I could have known sooner if my plant was going to die. Normally, I wait until the leaves look off, or are falling off. Either way, I wait for the plant to *show* in its appearance that something is wrong.

What I didn't know, is that root rot forms deep under the soil long before a plant shows any signs of growing pains.

The same goes for your child. Behavioural issues with your child means something is happening below the surface. Something is motivating your child to behave the way he does (and *no*, it's not attitude or evil intentions)!

A child does not choose to have behavioural issues just like a plant does not choose to have sick leaves. The plant grows within the environment provided, as does the child.

This section discusses age appropriate behaviours. This includes behaviours that may be challenging. You can understand your child when you understand what drives the behaviour. Understanding your child gives you strength, patience, and power. Power to support your child in his development.

Some behaviours can be found at certain stages of development. Other can span many age ranges. What we are seeing is mental health concerns showing up at younger ages than we are used to.

The difference is in the intensity felt by the child, especially during adolescence. The brain is much different during this time. This makes teen years emotional and tumultuous.

The information provided here is brief. It is not intended to replace the advice of medical or mental health professionals but to offer insight and guidance on your parenting journey.

LISTEN!

CHAPTER 13:

Birth to Eighteen Months of Age

"Any day spent with you is my favorite day,
so, today is my new favorite day."
- PIGLET

Your infant needs to know that you are going to be there. He is dependent on you to have his needs met. He needs food, clothing, shelter, and companionship to thrive.

Emotion is the primary source of communication at this age. It is the only way that your infant has to communicate. Problems arise when you lack patience or understanding of the infant language.

This is a challenging time for parents. Your child is dependent on you for his survival. Your child needs to trust you. When you tolerate the incessant emotional pining, he develops trust in you. Your tolerance communicates that his emotion is not too strong for you.

Your child needs you to be there. To *hold the space* for him. He needs to know that he matters enough for you to hear him. Even when he can't speak. Especially when he can't speak.

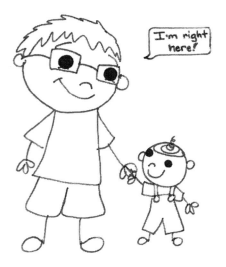

Spoiling

"Some people care too much. I think it's called love."
- WINNIE-THE-POOH

When I was a first-time parent, I was told to let my child cry. It was believed that crying was important to strengthen her lungs.

Good thing I prefer to trust my parenting instincts over popular belief.

Letting your child *cry it out* for their benefit is no longer popular belief. *Crying it out* programs the mind that no one is coming. That you are alone. That you don't matter.

Attending to your child's cries for help programs the mind that she matters. That she has value. That she is worth someone being there for her. Attending to your child's cries for help does not spoil your child.

You do not spoil a baby by attending to their needs. You communicate that someone is going to be there. That you are going to be there. This is where it all begins. This is when you help your child to know that they matter. That they have significance.

When you *hold the space* and are a firm bucket through sleepless nights and crying-filled days, your connection deepens. Trust develops. Trust that you will be there. Trust in you and trust in herself. That she can communicate and that she is capable to get her needs met.

LISTEN!

CHAPTER 14:
Eighteen Months to Three Years of Age

"The things that make me different are the things that make me me!"
- TIGGER

Your toddler is a miniature Indiana Jones. He is on an adventure to learn everything about his world. Your toddler stores all the information that he is learning during his quest. The more information he gathers, the more equipped he will be. He will use this information to guide his decisions for years to come.

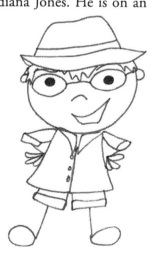

Unfortunately, toddlers are prone to getting in trouble. Parents often see the behaviour as wrong or bad. Your toddler does not know what 'bad' is.

Bad is often connected to behaviours that are inappropriate or unacceptable. You feel it is your duty to teach your toddler right from wrong.

Yes, we need to guide our children. Only, this is not what happens when we reprimand a toddler. What happens is that a toddler *learns* that *she* is bad. For your toddler, she was doing everything right. She was meeting her needs. Reprimands communicate that her *need* is wrong, that she is *wrong*. She cannot separate her behaviour from herself as a person.

This is when your child develops *shame*. She starts to believe that she is somehow defective. This is not your intent. You want to guide your child towards good decision making. So how do you guide your toddler's healthy exploration?

When your toddler's behaviour is an issue, *listen* to the need that is motivating the behaviour. Use LIVE. In this space, you empower your child to be part of the growing process. To make good decisions. You give her the gift of connecting to herself and her needs, and how to make helpful choices. This way, she grows in confidence and feels capable and strong.

CHAPTER 15:

Three to Six Years of Age

"People should seriously stop expecting normal from me.
We all know it's not going to happen."
- TIGGER

Your preschooler is on a mission. His mission is to prove that he is a superpower. He wants to be the superhero of your world. This is where he takes all that he has learned in his toddler days and works to make the world right.

He wants the world to be good. He associates negative experiences as wrong and positive experiences as right. Fairness is his mantra. He believes that he is good. So, he strongly believes that ALL his choices are good, or for the good of all people.

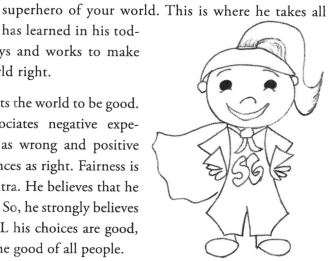

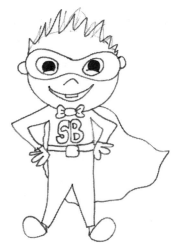

But, life is not fair, and right and wrong do not exist. You will teach your child the right and wrong, but this will differ from other people in his world. This is how your child will experience that the world is not fair. This experience will come with lots of emotion.

Your child will need you to support his own efforts to come up with ideas of how to run the world. He will need you to entertain his fantasies, even if you think they are crazy. When you do this, your child develops the ability to think for himself, to believe in himself, to trust himself.

Cultivate his ability to tolerate disappointment when others don't believe his fantasy. Foster trust in himself by nurturing the ability to feel his emotions and be okay.

Use LIVE to meet the challenging moments. Understand that his emotion serves a purpose. How you tend to his emotions determines his sense of self and his future success.

Oppositional Defiance

"Once in a while someone amazing comes along...
and here I am!"
- TIGGER

I casually walked into a high school one day and headed to the office to gather some information about a particular teenager. I was enthusiastically approached by a beloved support worker requesting some input into a personal situation. "My three-year-old grandson may be getting a diagnosis of oppositional defiant disorder and her parents are going crazy and don't know what to do!"

I was flabbergasted at the idea of a three-year-old being labelled as oppositional defiant. Oppositional Defiance (OD) is a behaviour disorder given to a child that may be exceptionally angry, defiant, or argumentative, just to name a few characteristics.

The intention of a three-year-old is to explore and master their world with your encouragement and support. I believe that in many cases, oppositional defiance is not an issue with the child, but with the way in which adults misread what the child's behaviour is communicating and the interactions that follow.

Oppositional defiance is when you have a child that actively defies doing what you want them to do. The definition of a three-year-old *is* oppositional defiance. A child at this age thinks they're a superhero, or some kind of powerful royalty. Naturally, you will get behaviours that include hearing the word *No* from your precious little one.

You may also hear the phrases, "You can't tell me what to do!" or "I hate you!" and have a child that delights in doing the opposite of what you ask.

It is tempting to focus on this behaviour to create change. After all, you are the parent. You could implement reprimands and consequences. You could demand that the behaviour change.

In these situations, the defiance may make sense to your child. But he can't find the words to express what is happening. Your child may be experiencing pent up negative energy. This may include feeling ignored. Feeling shut off from the world. Feeling unimportant and a need to prove his value.

Your child's behaviour is communicating. It's communicating anger, sadness, frustration, confusion. His behaviour is a protest against what I believe is a deep, intrinsic belief that is in all of us. That we are important.

Your child believes that he has value. The way the world interacts with him challenges this belief. And he has to challenge life back. Because what his behaviour is not communicating, is that he is bad.

So, what do you do with a child that is oppositional. A child that is defiant. Well, first you *listen*. Listen to what the behaviour is communicating. Is your child frustrated, sad, angry?

Then, hold your ground. Don't get pulled in to the emotion that surrounds defiant behaviour. When you do, you are functioning at the same level as your child. Use LIVE to help your child to feel heard and to get to a place where you can work through the behaviour together.

CHAPTER 16:

Six to 11 Years of Age

"As soon as I saw you,
I knew an adventure was going to happen."
WINNIE-THE-POOH

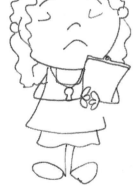

Your school-aged child has become a taskmaster. This is the age when your child is preparing their training manual for life. Your school-aged child likes to set goals, to make plans, and to lay out ground rules. This does not mean that your child will follow-through. Planning is the modus operandi.

It's like Lego. Children (and adults) spend more time building Lego than they do playing with it. It's in the building of the structure that they develop patience and perseverance.

Your school-age child is developing a sense of their position in the world. Social interactions are important to your child as she learns the social hierarchy. She may seem bossy or docile or both as she explores different characteristics. She is seeking safety and belonging.

To feel strong, she must feel connected to herself. This comes when you can stay solid in the midst of her emotional upheaval. You are on the path to sustainable emotional well-being.

Emotions will be high in moments of rejection. Use LIVE. When you help her navigate these emotional experiences, she will grow. This will help her to develop an understanding of what feels *right* to her, which is the only kind of right there is.

Screen Time

"Doing nothing often leads to the very best of something."
- WINNIE-THE-POOH

By now, you may have had difficulty with your child's screen time. We're bombarded with screens. We are told the detriments and the benefits of screen time. Your child may have become quite talented at arguing why their time in front of a screen time is the best thing for both of you.

Your child craves screen time because it provides a feeling of connection or belonging. It can offer a false sense of value, success or appreciation. There is a great amount of time and money invested to find out how to hook the mind of your child.

Screen time also satisfies a desire for stimulation or a distraction from stress. This may be misunderstood. The brain of a child needs time to have nothing stimulating it. The brain needs time of calm and peace.

When your child craves the screen, she is unsuccessfully using a machine to satiate needs. The problem is that a machine is not adequate to meet the needs of a child. It is a temporary distraction. They are needs that were intended to be met by an adult.

Your child needs social interaction for optimal development. Screens replace this social time by convincing us that it is effective. Companies invest in understanding how to keep your child engaged in their product.

To help you and your child, set boundaries and stick to them. Explain to your child ahead of time what the rules are. As your child gets older, reevaluate. Provide a rationale for changing the rules (because of age, season of the year, etc.) and keep ahead of the game.

You have to do what feels right for you and stick to it. Be consistent. Inconsistency is an invitation for your child to take control of the situation.

Be educated. There is a lot of information out there on how to guide the use of technology in your home. You can pretty much find evidence to support what you want to find. Ensure you know why you choose to do things the way that works for you and then set your boundaries. Your child will try to push the boundaries. Their development is contingent on sticking to your word.

Use LIVE. *Hold the space.* Keep your word and your child will develop her own ability to manage her disappointment, especially when it comes to screen time.

Bullying

"Hello Rabbit, Is that you?"
POOH

"Let's pretend it isn't" said RABBIT, *"and see what happens"*

It is popular belief that bullying is when someone is being hurt physically, emotionally, or mentally over an extended period of time. But bullying is more than that. Bullying is also about the feeling of belonging. We all want to belong.

Bullying is about pack mentality. Children choose to be a bystander, because it is safe. Being a bystander says that you belong. If your child had to choose between being a bully/bystander or being the child that is bullied, your child will choose the former.

If your child is being bullied, she could be experiencing depression, sadness, isolation, fear, nervousness, and hyper-vigilance. Behaviours may include school and activity refusal, or confusion. Wondering what she has done to upset the perpetrator. Taking the blame. Expressing things that are *wrong* with her, either appearance or characteristics.

Your child will be experiencing sadness and pain. She will feel insignificant, unwanted, defective, rejected, lonely. She may feel out of control inside and show a need for control outside.

If your child is the bully, she may play the victim. She may be unable to see herself as the problem. She will still be connected as part of a group, not isolated and more than one person on her side. She may also talk negatively or blame the victim.

Your child may be experiencing insecurity, a need for belonging, feeling out of control inside, and a need for control. Retaliation and a domino effect as hurt people hurt people.

When bullying occurs, children are needing to feel a sense of belonging. Children are trying to find out how they fit in their world.

A bully may target a child out of a need to feel like they belong. Belonging happens when a group targets one person due to a perceived weakness. This weakness commonly presents as emotional instability. So, the better your child can manage her emotions, the less likely she is to be bullied.

Cohesion of the group comes through a communal exclusion of the weak member. Think pack mentality. The pack supports the behaviour as togetherness strengthens the group.

A bully may also stem from internalized pain inflicted by another individual. The bully is acting out behaviour that is happening to her in an attempt to work through the pain. The bystander won't say anything. Their role is to support the leader. In doing so, this ensures their own belonging and safety within the group.

Generally, in a bullying situation, the victim is the isolated child or the child taking the blame. The child that is playing role of victim is often the perpetrator.

Boy bullying is more overt. The male social system is hierarchical with public displays of strength. "I am the best. I am stronger. I am smarter." These are normative to establish a healthy system of training and leadership towards manhood. The use of this system to hurt others physically, mentally, or emotionally is damaging.

Girl bullying is more covert. The girl world demands that everyone gets along. This becomes an issue when insecurity exists. A girl will mask this by using stories to defame another girl. She feels powerful when she can get others to believe her stories. She will even believe her own stories as the feeling of comradery is enticing and covers up the insecurity.

As a parent in a bullying situation, gather the facts. Do not jump to conclusions.

Build your child's emotional strength. Bullies prey on sensitive children as they appear weak. The key is not to hide your emotions, but to manage your emotions. When you are emotional, you give the bully power. If the bully is unable to affect your child, the bully will move on. Use LIVE. This is the source for your child in the face of a bully.

It is almost unanimous with the children I work with that the following things do not work and can make matters worse with a bully. This includes standing up to a bully. Pretending the bully does not exist (if the bully still affects your child). Telling a trusted adult. And the list goes on.

What does work, is building your child's emotional well-being so that the bully cannot have power over her. When your child is emotional, she is not in control. Help her to manage her emotions, and she will have control. Your child's unaffected emotional system will disarm the power of the bully.

Using LIVE will help your child to connect with her own emotions. When you *hold the space*, your child learns that she is capable of holding her own space. A bully preys on a child that can be emotionally activated. The strength that comes from using LIVE will become a protection from becoming a target for a bully.

ADHD and Learning Disabilities

"My spelling is wobbly. It's good spelling
— but it wobbles and the letters get in the wrong places."
- WINNIE-THE-POOH

ADHD is explained as an executive function disorder that contributes to attention, hyperactivity or impulsivity. But really, what is ADHD?

I have seen many learning assessments that identify areas of learning that are challenging for children. Many of these assessments give a diagnosis of ADHD. Some of these children have learning disabilities, and some do not. But all have an area where their learning is different.

There are three areas that can contribute to an ADHD diagnosis. They include hyperactivity, inattentiveness, and impulsivity. I find it interesting that these areas are similar to symptoms of someone that has experienced trauma.

Trauma is when the nervous system has been overloaded. This is much like a household fuse and electrical overload. Too much electricity surging through household wires causes the fuse to *blow*! Trauma is too much sensory input, or stressors, surging through the nervous system causing a person to *blow*!

When there is too much happening for the nervous system, the mind becomes overwhelmed and needs to respond.

So, take a child that has an area of weakness in his learning profile. Put this child in a classroom, or close proximity to peers. Place expectations on this child to *learn* in ways that do not work for the way his brain is designed. The child begins to *sense* that something isn't right. That something about *him* is not right.

Now add the fact that the most important thing for a child is to feel as if he belongs (remember the needs of the 0-18 month infant). This is a highly stressful situation for a child. With prolonged stress, the child will have difficulty focusing.

The mind is overwhelmed. Energy will be put into the survival of the child. This does not include doing well on a test. This includes making sure he notices every sound action going on around him. The child becomes inattentive, distracted, even hyperactive.

What if the child has a learning profile that states an inability to manage thought through memory or speed of understanding? Would this not lend to impulsivity?

You may think that I am simplifying a complex problem. The goal of this book is to provide a brief overview to help guide where to go from here. The point is that I see many children that have an ADHD diagnosis, but do not understand what is contributing to the symptoms.

There are children that have a neurological deficit that significantly inhibits their daily functioning. Some of these children have a diagnosis that includes a deficit in the mental processes that underly the way a child learns, aka, a learning disability.

A child with learning challenges lives in a world that expects more than the child can adequately accomplish. A child is stressed when you expect more than the child can do. Especially when the child has put forth adequate effort. The result is a stressed child.

And what happens to your stressed-out child. Your child can not focus. Your child will act out. Your child will feel sad, frustrated, stressed!

What is important here is to understand your child. Your child knows himself and needs you to learn how to know him. Difficulties may include managing the way their mind integrates the world, difficulty in managing schoolwork or social encounters, a felt sense of difference from peers, a feeling of incompetence.

If your child has a psychoeducational assessment, it is important to understand the numbers and what that means for your child. To understand your child's strengths and build on this. To see ADHD as a diagnosis, not an explanation. And to learn how to understand your child.

Here is what is happening for your child. His brain does not work in the same way as the average child. Children can struggle to communicate this to an adult. Your child's stress may increase their learning challenges. Stressed children cannot focus.

Here is what you can do. Understand your child separate from the diagnosis. Your child is more than the boxes that define a diagnosis. Seek to understand your child's patterns and non-verbal communications. Communicate understanding by *listening*.

Remove sources of stress. A stressed child is not a happy child. If school is a stress, understand how your child learns. Don't blame behaviour on the diagnosis. Support strengths and acknowledge the challenges.

If your child has a psychoeducational assessment, seek to understand the data. Understand how your child learns or does not learn. Help him to understand what has led to the behaviours that have led to a diagnosis. Empower your child with the parts of him that he knows make him feel capable. We all have those parts and it feels great when others point them out.

Have realistic expectations. Understand the difference between choice and challenge. Your child choosing not to do something is different from feeling incapable. Your child may feel like they keep putting in their best effort with no success. You can imagine how deflating this is!

Remember, your child wants to please you and win your praise. If they struggle to do this, they are hurting inside. They want to be a success and they need you to know them, to believe in them, and to support them to get there. Using LIVE will help to bring a connection between the two of you. Your child will finally feel that he is understood.

Anxiety

> *"Some people talk to animals.*
> *Not many listen, though. That's the problem."*
> - WINNIE-THE-POOH

Anxiety is a prolonged state of activation of the nervous system. This may include nervousness, school refusal, an incessant need to be close to a parent, sleep disturbances, irritability, worry, apprehension, and the list goes on...

This behaviour is communicating fear of sensations that occur in the body and the associated feeling of discomfort. The nervous system processes stimuli as threatening and is unable to shut itself off.

The body is in a continued activated state. The mind becomes suspicious of any incoming stimuli. The mind believes that it needs to be in a constant state of protection.

When your child is anxious, validate the fear. Be with the emotion. You may think the situation is silly or unwarranted. Fair enough. But your expression of this will only make the anxiety worse.

Make the fear matter of fact. Stay neutral. Your child will look to you for how to be with the situation. Don't give it more energy but be respectful of the energy that is there. Remember, this comes from the Emotional Brain. It demands an audience. All you need to do is to *listen* and it will start to settle a bit. Slow, gradual exposure can help your child to overcome some fears, if you *listen* and LIVE.

Depression

> *Thanks for noticin' me.*
> - EEYORE

Depression is an extended duration of feeling low energy and an inability to engage with life as usual. This may include difficulty sleeping and feelings of fatigue, guilt, feeling insignificant and hopeless, irritable, contentious, loss of appetite, despondent, and much more...

His behaviour is communicating internalized anguish and exhaustion due to fighting an internal or external battle.

Depression is anger turned inwards. It includes a tendency to take blame on oneself, or an inability to feel capable of being yourself. The mind feels exhausted after suffering for an extended period of time. The mind and body have shut down and is rebooting.

What you can do for your child is to *listen*. Listening is the fastest way to help your child to feel connected to you and connected to himself. Talking with another person that listens is validating.

It is okay to be sad. It is normal to be sad. It is not normal to be low for an extended period of time. If you are experiencing any of the above, get help for you so that you can help your child. Being there for your child is a powerful stimulant for change.

Use LIVE to validate where your child is at. When you validate the pain, the mind begins to heal. Her connection with you will grow. Her strength will grow when you are present with her internalized pain.

CHAPTER 17:

12 to 18 Years of Age

"People say nothing is impossible, but I do nothing every day."
- WINNIE-THE-POOH

If you had the chance, would you go back to your teen years? Those days of feeling misunderstood, stressed, confused, lonely. This has got to be one of the most misunderstood times of life. Here is some insight that might help.

Around age 12, the adolescent brain goes through a re-modelling process in preparation for adulthood. This change takes about 12 years. At 12, your child begins the transition. You start to notice the change in behaviours or reactivity. The brain will actually feel a bit like it did when your child was about 2-4 years old. They will feel emotionally raw.

Ages 13-15 have got to be the hardest in terms of feeling dark, lonely, lost, empty. These are all normal processes for this age group. We just don't realize that and tend to treat this normal experience as a problem.

What your child needs is emotional support. What your child does not need is rejection, criticism, or demands on their behaviour. Your child *looks* older. But, he feels like a helpless two-year-old on the inside.

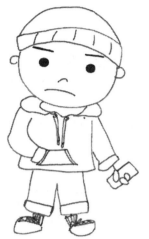

To add to this is all that hormonal action going on inside their bodies. For girls, they begin the monthly cycle and waves of emotions that accompany this. This is not the cause of the behaviour, as there are many other developmental processes taking place. But, it is a contributor.

The boys don't have it any easier. From the time of puberty, boys have an average of four surges of testosterone a day. Every day. For the rest of their lives. This makes boys have random moments throughout the day where they feel an overwhelming need to move energy through their body. This can come out as physical aggression, or other forms of outward behaviour.

Male or female, this is a time of raw emotion and exploration.

Your child will no longer be willing to listen to your parental wisdom. No matter how perfect and wonderful your child may be, your teen will reject any advice or opinion you offer. The rejection is not a choice. It's an instinctive response from the mind of a teenager. This instinct is to prepare him for independence.

You will have more success when you present your suggestions as options. You also provide the consequences and how the decisions will play out. Then, you back off and leave the decision making to your teen. You also need to be comfortable with your teen making mistakes. Mistakes are great! Mistakes make the best teachers.

Your teen will make mistakes. This is how they learn. They have the ability to make good decisions when the brain is in the right frame of mind. But the teenage brain is an Emotional Brain. The brain is restructuring during adolescence. For the earlier teen years, their brain acts much like it did when your teen was two years old.

When emotions come into play, use LIVE. Teenage emotions are intense, and they need you to *hold the space* for them. They need this now more than at any other time in their life. When you do this, they feel secure. They feel strength. They feel capable. Their mind re-corrects and can go to a place of problem solving. This is the best way to prepare your child for adulthood.

As parents, we want to help with the problem solving. We have years of experience making bad decisions. With all our wisdom, we want to protect our children from emotional harm.

We also want to protect ourselves from emotional harm. If our children listen to us, they won't have to hurt. Which means, we won't have to hurt.

It's guaranteed that you are going to hurt. Your teen has to experience hurt to grow.

Your role is not to do the problem solving for your child. Your role is to help them to manage their emotions so they can grow. We must give our children space to learn for themselves. We can be available to guide them if they ask for our help. They won't ask if they don't trust you.

You gain their trust by giving them space. By trusting that they will make the right decision, or that they will grow through their mistakes. Your role is to help them through the process of managing their emotions. Because, when your teen can manage his emotions, he can handle anything.

There is another misunderstanding about teenagers. We tend to think that teens are moody. We treat this as a problem. This is not a problem; this IS the definition of adolescence.

The teenage brain is emotional. The Thinking Brain is re-modelling, like a kitchen upgrade. The cupboards and the sink are still there, but the kitchen is getting new flooring and new appliances. Teenagers are emotional because their Emotional Brain is more active, especially between the ages of 13-15.

Your teen will feel alone, dark, empty, and lost. This is not a problem; this is an opportunity. This is Mother Nature's gift for your child to get to know herself. It is in this void that she experiences tolerance; tolerance for the emotions that come with being human.

A child needs support through this time. She needs to know that this is normal. She needs support to not be afraid of the growth that occurs. This is possible when our child's emotions do not scare us. Then we help our child, so their emotions don't scare them.

As adults, this scares us if we have not faced our own void. The void is not to be feared. The void is the space where we learn that we can make it. We have good days. We have bad days. Emotions are cyclical. We grow through our emotions.

Be the bucket for your teenager. Expect that they will be emotional. If you need a bucket, seek this out through friends, family or professionals. Do what you need to do so that you can *hold the space* for your child as she grows through the emotions of adolescence.

And one last thing. If you say, "I understand!" to your teenager, she will shut you out. Why? because she doesn't even understand herself, so how could you understand her. She develops this understanding through managing her emotions.

Use LIVE to help her connect to herself. She will grow in strength and will be on the path to emotional well-being.

Self-Harm

> *"When stuck in the river, it is best to dive and swim to the bank yourself before someone drops a large stone on your chest in an attempt to hoosh you there."*
> - EEYORE

Self-harm is when you hurt yourself on purpose, but you do not plan to kill yourself. The harm can be physical, emotional, or mental. Self-harm can happen with kids as young as five or six. It has become a popular form of dealing with pain.

Self-harm may include cutting, scratching, or digging sharp objects into the skin. Often found on the upper or lower arms, the thighs, and the stomach, banging the head on hard surfaces, hitting the head with the hand, substance misuse, sleep deprivation, pulling hair out or cutting off hair at the root, or biting oneself.

If your child is self-harming, she is in emotional pain. The programming of the mind is for survival. The mind moves you away from pain. If your child is hurting herself, the mind believes this will feel better than the current state of pain.

Self-harm provides relief. When you create pain on the body, the body releases a pain killer to protect the mind from the inflicted pain. A numbing occurs for roughly 5-20 minutes. During this time, your child experiences a temporary moment of relief.

Self-harm helps your child to feel. After an extended period of suffering, your child can become disconnected from herself. The mind craves a re-connection. Self-inflicted pain confirms that your child can still feel. It conveys that she still exists and produces the sensation of ability to feel again.

To help your child, stay calm. Create a boundary of safety. Show that you can *hold the space* by not engaging with her emotions. Use LIVE to guide you. Attend to your own fears, but do not make them the center of the situation. Your child needs to know that you can be the bucket when her own emotions are feeling out of control.

It will help if you DO NOT blame yourself. DO NOT reprimand, threaten, or punish your child. This is you attending to your emotional needs, not hers. Any attempt to control what is happening is to satiate your own fear, anger, or embarrassment.

Do not try to solve the problem. Whatever is affecting your child has been going on for some time. Listen to your child. If your child is not talking to you they are afraid of your response. They don't trust that you can manage your own emotions. She needs you to hold your space to help her to grow within her own.

Self-harm is a symptom of pain. Your child is craving closeness, connection and belonging. The way back to connection with herself and with you is to start with LIVE.

Suicide

> *"Don't blame me if it rains"*
> - EEYORE

Suicide is when you want to die. You think about it, or you plan to make it happen.

Thoughts include, "I am going to/want to kill myself!", "I don't want to live/to be here anymore!", "I want to die!", "I shouldn't be here anymore!", "It would solve everything if I wasn't here anymore.", "I can't do it anymore."

When someone is suicidal, they are communicating a feeling of overwhelming pain. If you hear these words from your child, it translates to, "I am in so much pain and I need a way to make it stop. I need a way out!"

Children exist in the moment, even a teenager (until the later teen years). The mind is searching for a solution to the current level of pain and the source of the pain. Not being here is a great solution.

Your child is feeling desperation. Your child feels like there is no other solution. They may still be thinking in black and white. Your child's Thinking Brain is not yet functional enough to consider other options and is existing in the moment.

Your child is experiencing confusion. Your child craves connection and belonging. If a child is talking about wanting to die, they are feeling disconnected from you or from himself. Something deep inside says he has value, but his world does not confirm this.

Your child is also experiencing blame. He feels like he is the problem. He feels helpless and that there is no other option.

To support your child, stay calm. Create a boundary of safety. Show that you can *hold the space* by not engaging with his emotions. Use LIVE to guide you. Attend to your own fears, but do not make them the center of the situation.

Ask your child the question, if we could make the pain go away, would you still want to die? Often suicide is a matter of getting the pain to stop. Your child needs help to tolerate the pain that is within.

If the emotions are intolerable, find professional help that can heal the pain.

If this is too hard for you, get help for you so you can be there for your child. You can get help for your child but getting help for you will do more in the long run. He wants you. He needs you. He needs your strength. If you need help strengthening your bucket, find a bucket for you. Then be the strong bucket for your child.

Use LIVE. It lets your child know that you *hear* him. It helps your child to reconnect to himself, and then to reconnect to you. That is the core of what we all seek. A strong connection to oneself, and a strong connection to others. You provide the beginning of that wonderful journey.

LISTEN!

PART E:
BONUS PARENTING
HACKS

W e all need a little help from time to time. Parenting is not easy, especially in today's world.

The parenting hacks presented in this section include a number of tactics that I developed over time. Many of these hacks were the result of using LIVE and working with my child for the purpose of growth and development. This is my toolbox for raising a child.

When my daughter was 16, she said, "Mom, you know what makes you a good parent? You apologize. But you don't just say you're sorry. You actually listen and try to understand what you may have done wrong. And then you go to work to fix it to make it all better."

Another important aspect in child rearing is to keep your word. I learned how important this was by seeing the affect this had on my children. When I kept my word, they appeared to feel safer, stronger.

My kids knew this. I watched so many parents *count to 5*, do nothing about it, and see the negative effect on their child. I was not going to be that parent.

So, I counted down: 3-2-1...0. I think we only ever got to zero once, because my child knew I meant business. Zero was always an immediate consequence that was small but significant. I used this sparingly. You have to be smart in the chess game of child rearing. Kids are very clever.

But it's more than smarts! Children are very attuned to their parents. You're their source of survival. So naturally, your child will be able to read your every move. Why do you think your child can so easily drive you crazy? Because they're are an extension of you.

From the mouth of babes, we can learn our greatest lessons. Here are some of mine.

CHAPTER 18:
Pre-loading

Tell your child beforehand what you plan to do.

Imagine you became inspired by a *Mission Impossible* movie. You decided that you wanted to jump out of an airplane. In preparation, you do a training session to ensure your safety and survival.

Parenting is not much different from jumping out of an airplane. You take a giant leap with a general plan, but not sure exactly how the journey will unfold. Pre-loading is a way to ensure your emotional safety and survival.

One of your greatest tactics for smooth parenting is to be preventative. Pre-loading is an effective strategy to prevent an emotional eruption in the home. Pre-loading offers household rules, guidelines, and consequences. You present these to your child beforehand, so when the time comes, there is no debate.

When you plan ahead of time, your child will know what to expect. It will be easier for you to remain neutral when your child loses it. She will *lose it*. You will see a tantrum of sorts as your child will push the boundary. They do this to grow. They need you to stick to your word for the growth process to be complete.

When you go back on your word, you teach your child that you are weak. Either you were weak at planning, or you were too weak to withstand their emotional prowess. This makes your child feel uneasy deep within. They need your boundary structure to instill a sense of safety.

You also teach your child that they are not valuable. Your child feels important when you stick to your word, even if they are spouting profanities at you. Keeping your word AND your cool is powerful. This communicates that she is special, important, powerful and it will make her want to be like you.

The emotions of your child serve a purpose. To communicate discomfort or disappointment and to get you to change your mind. This does not come from a place of manipulation but from a need to stop the discomfort of disappointment.

Imagine the strength you will give to your child if you help them to tolerate disappointment. Imagine how this will help your child through life and all the decisions that your child will face.

Whining, pleading, and bargaining are attempts to get you to defend your position. When you engage in defending yourself, this gives your child power and fuels their plight. You become exhausted and tired and consider giving in. DON'T. Otherwise, their system wins, and it is not strength promoting. Giving in is strength suffocating.

Hold the space.

Over time, your child will grow in her ability to manage the discomfort of emotion. Let the system work it through while you stay firm and present. Pre-load, let her know ahead of time and arm yourself to stay strong. Tell her this is for her growth because she matters to you. This is the path to emotional well-being, and you are the cultivator.

LISTEN!

CHAPTER 19:
Yes/Maybe/No

"I would have liked for it to go on a while longer."
- WINNIE-THE-POOH

Ever feel exhausted by all the constant badgering by your child? Yes/Maybe/No is how to maximize parenting effectiveness while minimizing your efforts.

When your child has a request, your answer will be *yes, maybe,* or *no.*

If your answer is "Yes!" it's his lucky day.

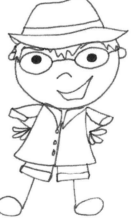

If your answer is *maybe*, he has some work to do. This is an invitation to present evidence that will sway your decision in their favor. This also buys you time to make a decision that you will stick with.

If your answer is *no*, they are out of luck. You only choose this when you have a definite rationale and your will not go back on your word.

It is very important that you never go back on your word. This gains trust. It makes it easier on you the next go-around. When you prove that you won't change your answer, your child will spend less energy trying to do so.

Take the time you need to make the response you will stick with.

When *no* is the answer, give a reason. Provide space for a discussion with a reminder that your decision is firm. When your child pushes for you to change your answer, reiterate the *no* and remind him that the discussion is over.

Your child will try to engage you in conversation. He will poke and prod to get you to defend yourself. When this happens, you fuel the debate. The discussion ends at *no*. Your child gets two responses and that is all the energy you need to give to the discussion. You can invite your child to do all the begging and bartering he would like, but you will not be part of that.

Story

Timmy sat himself on the floor. While playing with Lego, he started his quest for a large popcorn at the movies that afternoon.

Timmy: "Can I get a large popcorn at the movies today?"

Nana: "No, a small is big enough."

Timmy: "Pleaaase! I'm so hungry!" (Triggering the caregiver's responsibility to provide).

Nana: "I will feed you before you go."

Timmy: "Pleaaase! You never let me get a large popcorn (triggering parent's guilt)".

Nana: "You got a medium the last time you went and that was enough."

Timmy: (Now rolling on the floor). "But you never let me do this and this is a special occasion and…"

Nana was ready to respond. I stopped her. I shared that defending her position provides energy to the child. Engaging in the discussion provides hope to your child that you might give in. If he does it long enough, you will tire and change your mind. That is the purpose of begging.

So, don't engage. Preload and set the ground rules for how you will respond to requests. Then, be consistent and stick to your word.

LISTEN!

CHAPTER 20:
The Physical Boundary:
When Your Child is Physical

"Watch me scare the stripes off of this imposter."
- TIGGER

For some children, the answer "No" is an invitation to become a hellion. Use the following guide for a child that becomes physical.

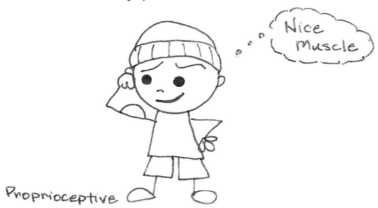

Let your child know the following rules for your home. When upset, there is no hurting yourself, hurting others, or hurting objects.

Let your child know that when any of the points on the list occur, that the following will happen.

If you are stronger than your child, you put your arms around her. You do not hold too loose so that she can get free, and you do not hold too tight so that she cannot move around.

Your child is craving this! Your child needs to know that someone can keep them safe when they feel out of control.

This is holding the space. Literally. Your child is feeling scared of herself. She will yell things at you that will hurt your heart, but ignore this. You have to remain calm. You have to physically be the bucket to provide a sense of safety to her Emotional Brain.

Do this until she calms, until she breaks free, or until she can agree to not hurting herself, others, or things.

If your child is stronger than you, let her know that if any of the above occurs, you will call the police. Stick to your word. All it takes is following through on a call to the police and the behaviour will change. If it does not, seek outside support.

Caveat: To expect your child to never become physical, you must not be physical yourself.

CHAPTER 21:
How to Get Your Child to Do Just About Anything

"Life. It's not about how fast you run or how high you climb, but how well you bounce."
- TIGGER

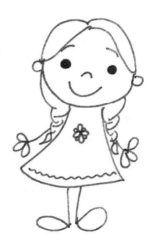

Much like *yes/maybe/no,* you only have to say something twice. Your days of saying,

"I've told you 10 times already!" are over.

Saying anything more than twice is too much effort. Here are five steps to get your child to complete a task.

1. One, determine what it is that you want completed. You want her room cleaned.

2. Two, make sure she understands all the steps involved. For you, cleaning her room means that she makes her bed, her clothes are in the laundry and the floor is clear. To your daughter, this means that junk gets pushed under the bed and the blankets cover the pillow.

   Make sure that your child understands the steps that you want done. Teach her. Make a list. Make sure that it is age appropriate expectation.

3. Three, provide choices. Give her some space to get it done by providing choice. "I will take you to the pool/your friend's house when your room is clean. You have until 5:00. It's now 1:00.

4. Four, establish a bargaining chip. So, you can choose if you want to go sooner or later. You must clean your room before I will drive you.

5. Five, follow through. Be prepared to drive her as soon as her room is clean. Don't make her wait as you want to reinforce the self-motivation. If she doesn't clean her room until 4:59, let her know that she chose not to go to the pool/friend's house. Remind her that you left it to her to get the task done at her leisure.

You are doing your part to show that you care by keeping your word. If she gets upset, you can help her see how she chose anger and put herself in that situation. You can add that you are looking forward to the next time that she may make a decision that will make her happy.

You can also offer to assist if she wants to review what may have gotten in the way of completing the task. This is to help the next time this happens, not to get you to give in. Stick to your word and she will start to take more ownership.

Your child WILL test you to see if you will keep your word. This is about trust and safety. If your child can trust you to be flaky, they will feel unsafe, weak and scared. If your child can trust you to be consistent, they will feel safer and stronger.

Timmy: "You're a #$%^."

Grampa: "If you talk to me like that again, I will not talk to you for the remainder of the day."

Timmy: "Well, you're a #%$^@ ^&* $%^&."

Grampa: "This is the second and last warning. If you speak to me like that again, I won't be talking to you for the rest of the day."

Timmy: "I don't care, you're a @%#% #$%^ @#$%& #$%&*&."

Grampa didn't talk to Timmy for the rest of the day. Timmy tried everything throughout the day to get Grandpa to engage. Grampa knew that Timmy's survival brain would try everything possible to get a response; he would find the most sensitive area to get Grandpa dysregulated and subsequently engage with Timmy's system. (Remember the picture of the ant being stepped on)!

Grampa did not give in and the remainder of the week was free of any rude language directed towards Grandpa.

Boundary setting with love is what your child's system craves! It is what he needs to grow towards maturation and independence.

LISTEN!

CHAPTER 22:
Realistic Expectations

"This isn't working out the way I was hoping."
- TIGGER

Your child is still a child. They do not have the experiences that you have had to influence the way they look at the world. They understand the world through their limited experiences. Try to understand your child through the way he sees the world.

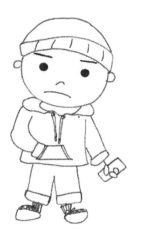

You expect great things from your child. You want their room spotless or the dishes done without reminders.

How good are you at keeping up with your tasks? If you struggle to keep your room clean, don't expect the same from your child. We often put our pressures on our child instead of setting them up for success. They need coaching and guidance.

Have you ever felt frustrated, misunderstood, and undervalued? If only you could see through their eyes.

Try to understand your child. *Listening* to your child does not mean that they get their way, or that they have power over you. *Listening* is a way to feel understood. It's empowering for you and your child when you step back and hear him.

Story

My tenacious daughter was an independent three-year-old. She preferred to walk on the busy street near our home without holding onto my hand. "I can do it all by myself" was one of the first sentences to come out of her mouth!

I provided constant reminders to stay between the white lines when we came to a crosswalk. Without fail, like a tightrope walker, she would balance herself right on the white line. I would remind her to remain *between* the white lines, and she persisted in her position on the white line.

Years later, when my daughter was about the age of 19, I told her this story. Shockingly she replied, "Mom, I thought that when you said to stay between the white lines, that you meant walk on the white line and don't go off of them."

ALL THOSE YEARS OF THINKING SHE WAS DEFIANT AND SHE WAS JUST BEING OBEDIENT.

How many other moments were misunderstood and informed years of mis-labelling my child?

Listen to your child. Again, all they want is to feel close to you and to please you. They need you! If your child is upsetting you and pushing buttons, you may be misunderstanding what they are communicating.

Story

I had a mom come into my office with her 10-year-old that was acting out. "This is only happening at home" was the exacerbated concern. After spending time together, I deduced that he wasn't feeling connected and that was all he was wanting. Mom turned to the son and said, "I think we are pretty connected, don't you?" The son quickly shook his head.

Even when we think we are doing a good enough job, our children may *see* things differently. Be open to how they perceive and see the world. Remember they are not a little you, they are a little them!

LISTEN!

CHAPTER 23:

Sleeplessness

"When all else fails, take a nap."
- WINNIE-THE-POOH

Children are like sponges and spend their days learning about the world. They take in enormous amounts of information during the day.

At nighttime, the brain shuts down all its parts to reboot for the coming day. All its parts, that is, except the Emotional Brain.

The Emotional Brain remains active to make sure that you are protected from danger. This is why you have a harder time sleeping in an unfamiliar hotel or anywhere away from home. Because the Emotional Brain remains online and active, just in case there is any danger lurking.

Any emotional disturbances felt during the day by your child will be front and center in your child's mind. Any unresolved emotional disturbances from the past could be front and center in your child's mind. As your child lays in bed, their Emotional Brain is cycling threw these raw emotions.

Thoughts go round and round as the Thinking Brain tries to find a solution. This can be overwhelming.

To deny the emotion is to make it bigger. Telling your child to go to sleep, there are no monsters, everything is okay, will make the fear stronger. You are not acknowledging the message of the Emotional Brain. So, the feeling intensifies.

Use LIVE to take away some of the power of the Emotional Brain. This may help your child to come to a solution, or just alleviate some of the emotional pressure. Be prepared as this will take time, and it will be late. But when you invest the time, eventually, the pressure valve is released, and the power that drives the behaviour will melt away.

Use LIVE to calm the brain somewhat and then you can agree to talk about the situation in the morning.

CHAPTER 24:
Rewind

*"Love is taking a few steps backward, maybe even more...
to give way to the happiness of the person you love."*
- WINNIE-THE-POOH

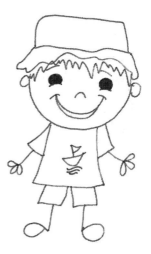

Rewind is a technique that I use when a child needs to change their behaviour. I also use this when I need to change the way that I may have behaved.

Rewind is when you go back and do it all over again. But this time, you substitute the desired behaviour in the place of what was unwanted.

I often use this when my children have a conflict, like when they start to get worked up and say things that are hurtful.

I first have them stop and take space until they are in a better place. Next, without letting time elapse, we go back to the time just before the situation started to get bad. Then I have them go through the scenario again, only this time, they have to use different words or behaviours. They have to make the situation amicable and reestablish the strong relationship that they have.

Your children start yelling and swearing at each other. You tell them it must stop. If they don't, you get one to leave the room or whatever it takes to make the situation halt. Once they have calmed down, you bring everyone together and describe the behaviour that you want changed.

The next time a moment is unacceptable, for you or your child, you can change the story. You can generate new habits. It's like erasing a sketch and redrawing the lines the way that you want them.

You have the power to create the sketches of life that you want for your home and your family. It all starts with you.

CHAPTER 25:

Mistakes

"Always watch where you are going. Otherwise, you may step on a piece of the forest that was left out by mistake."
- POOH'S LITTLE INSTRUCTION BOOK

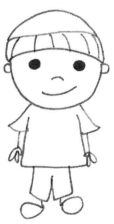

Expect that you will mess up. That's a realistic expectation and a good thing. Mistakes are a part of life, especially the life of a parent. The good news is that being a parent is all about learning from your mistakes.

It takes strength and humility to own up to your mistakes. This can have a powerful effect on your child. Children are very forgiving. When you mess up, you provide a wonderful teaching tool for your child.

LISTEN!

One of the greatest teaching tools for your child is to apologize. A sincere apology is taking ownership of whatever it is that you have done that you or your child would like to change.

The following is 5 steps to a sincere apology.

One, ask permission to apologize. This shows respect for their space and makes them feel valued and important.

Two, show understanding that you have caused them to hurt.

Three, present a plan to fix what you have done.

Four, include how you will not repeat what you did (otherwise, the apology is nullified).

Five, talk it through and then ask for forgiveness.

Your child's ability to manage their emotions comes from you! How you manage and model your own internal disruptions provides a blueprint for your child. You cannot expect a behaviour from your child unless you have modeled that behaviour yourself. Take ownership. Find strength in knowing that you can grow together. The result is a strong bond with your child, and your child's strong bond with themselves.

"It is not what you do, but what you do after what you've done." - Brandys Evans

"It is not what you do, but what you do after what you've done."
- BRANDYS EVANS

CONCLUSION

"If the person you are talking to doesn't appear to be listening, be patient. It may simply be that he has a small piece of fluff in his ear."
- WINNIE -THE-POOH

I remember a time when my daughter was four. She sat behind me as I drove along Grand Boulevard on the North Shore. Her brother sat within arms' reach, perfectly positioning himself for her taunting.

The shrill cry of my little guy launched me into parenting mode. We were on our way to Gramma and Grampa's house. We didn't have a television at the time, but the grandparents did. So, I presented the consequence. There would be no TV once we arrived at our destination.

I continued to drive. Quiet on the outside, but tormented on the inside. My quietude was an attempt to keep my word and not show a bluff. But I was fretting inside. Would she think that I was a terrible parent and hate me? My tenacious daughter was silent. 'What was she thinking?' was the thought that ran through my head.

Even though the silence was a result of my internal conflict, it turned out to be a blessing. This allowed the space for my daughter to reflect on the experience. What unfolded next was one of my greatest learning experiences.

When we arrived, I saw the focus of my daughter's silence. She presented me with a piece of paper. The paper had over 50 hearts on it. In the center were the words, *I Love You, Mom*. And in her eyes was the look of hope. Hope that I would be receptive and accepting. That I would fill her hurt heart with love.

What I learned in that moment was that a child needs boundaries. Boundaries, placed with love, communicate. Boundaries communicate to a child that they matter. This communication happens *at their core.* At their core is where they learn that they are significant. That they are valued.

When you communicate this to a child, without the use of any words at all, a child grows. A child feels invincible, capable, and powerful. Powerful enough to make things happen.

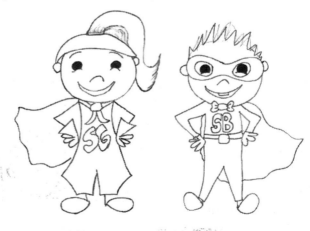

In the first section of this book, you learned about the different parts of the brain. Understanding the role of each part of the brain will help you to understand the role of emotion in your child's life. You help your child to manage their emotions when you understand how and why these parts of the brain work together to keep your child safe.

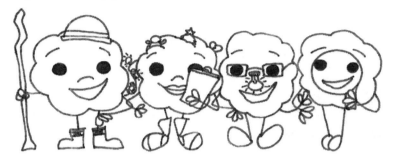

In the second section of this book, you learned about emotion. We broke it down to help provide clarity about how the mind and body keep us safe. This information provides compassion for the process of emotion. And emotion serves the purpose of keeping us alive.

In the third section of this book, you learned how to grow your child's ability to regulate emotion. You also learned how self-regulation connects your child to you. And when your child is connected to you, she can connect to herself. The result is a happy child and a happy you.

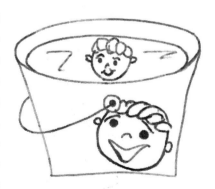

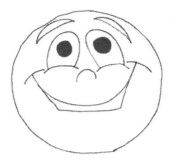

In the fourth section of the book, you learned what you can expect of your child during the different stages of development. You also learned that your child does not want to be bad or *challenging*. You learned about how behaviour comes from trying to meet a need. When you understand what is driving the behaviour, you understand your child.

In the fifth section, you are provided with parenting interventions that foster strength and growth. When followed, life will go a bit more smoothly, with less emotion. Not easier, but smoother.

This book is the result of years of learning, from my children, and from the countless parents and children that I have served and worked with.

The concepts in this book will bring you closer to your child and closer to yourself. It really is quite easy, it's just not what we are used to. Listen to your child. Listen to you. Don't be afraid of the discomfort that comes from within. And don't let it take over and run your world. This is simply a gift. An opportunity to *hear*. An opportunity to grow.

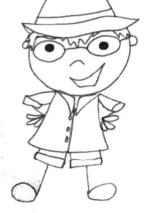

We spend so much time being afraid of discomfort. We are afraid of feeling pain. But pain is our source of growth. Go into the pain with your child. Identify the emotion that they are feeling and just stay with it. It will be there briefly, and then it will pass.

Just like a rain cloud that comes in, dumps out its moisture, and passes on. The emotion won't last. When you can help your child to be with the emotion, your child's tolerance will increase. As his tolerance increases, he can manage his emotions. He can manage the stressors that come his way now and in the future.

Validate the emotion. Let him know that it is okay to feel the way he does. And then show that you get it. That you can see why he responded the way he did (even if you don't agree).

When you do this, your child will feel strong. He will feel capable. He will thrive. He will be connected to himself. He will be connected to you.

"But it isn't easy," said Pooh. "Because Poetry and Hums aren't things which you get, they're things which get you. And all you can do is to go where they can find you."
-WINNIE-THE-POOH

When you *get* your child, they will give you their heart. Then you can help them to manage their own heart and then be strong all on their own.

LISTEN!

INVITATION: If you *heard* this book *speak* to you, I would encourage you to share the book and it's contents with anyone that interacts with children, including parents, grandparents, teachers, best friends, child support workers, and coaches, so we can raise generations of strong individuals.

For any questions or comments, please contact me at info@brandysevans.com brandysevans.com @brandysevans

If you would like to support the contents of the book, please consider leaving a review.

Go to www.brandysevans.com/free-download to receive your free guide to LISTEN! Helping Your Child Manage Their Emotions.

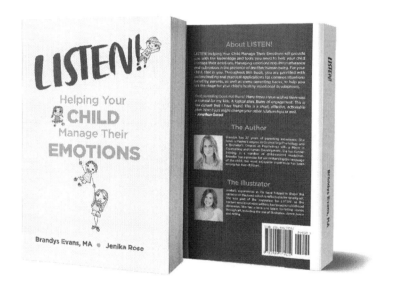

Manufactured by Amazon.ca
Bolton, ON

11417465R00103